American Academy of Orthopaedic Surgeons

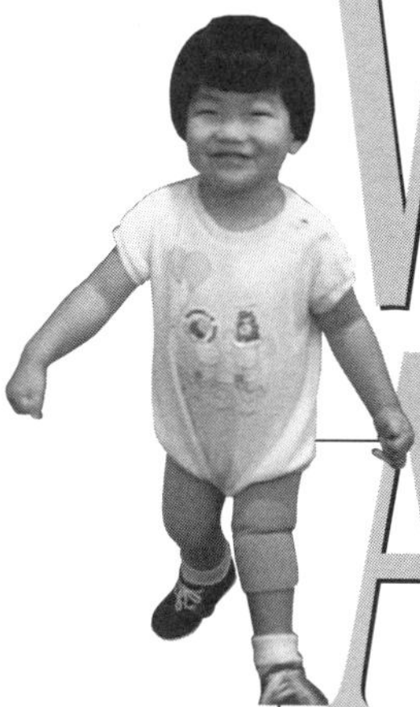

Who Is Amelia?

Caring for Children With Limb Deficiencies

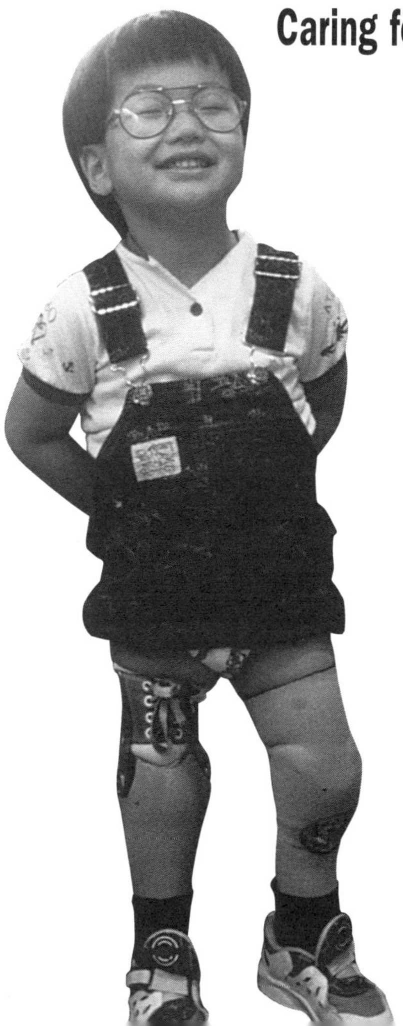

Hugh G. Watts, MD

Clinical Professor, Orthopaedics

University of California, Los Angeles

Shriners Hospital for Crippled Children

Los Angeles, California

Mary Williams Clark, MD

Chief, Division of Pediatric Orthopaedics

Department of Orthopaedic Surgery

Medical College of Ohio

Toledo, Ohio

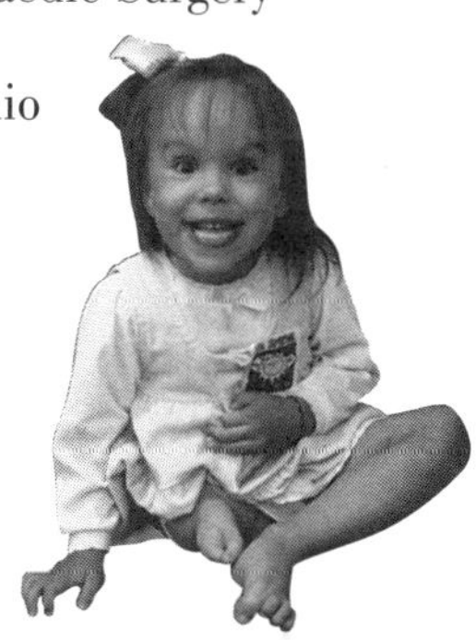

Staff

Marilyn L. Fox, PhD
Director, Department of Publications

Loraine Edwalds
Production Manager

Pamela Hutton Erickson
Art Direction and Design

Published 1998
by the American Academy of Orthopaedic Surgeons
6300 North River Road
Rosemont, Illinois 60018
1-800-626-6726

The Academy has made the material presented in *Who Is Amelia?* available for educational purposes only. This material is not intended to present the only, or necessarily best, methods or procedures for the medical situations discussed, but rather is intended to represent an approach, view, statement, or opinion of the author(s) or producer(s), which may be helpful to others who face similar situations.

Some drugs or medical devices demonstrated in Academy courses or described in Academy print or electronic publications have not been cleared by the Food and Drug Administration (FDA) or have been cleared for specific uses only. The FDA has stated that it is the responsibility of the physician to determine the FDA clearance status of each drug or device he or she wishes to use in clinical practice.

Furthermore, any statements about commercial products are solely the opinion of the author(s) and do not represent an Academy endorsement or evaluation of these products. These statements may not be used in advertising or for any commercial purpose.

Printed in the U.S.A.

ISBN 0-89203-179-4

Table of Contents

Preface

Dear Reader:

Who are you? This manual was written with the focus on teaching orthopaedic residents the special needs of children who are amputees or are born with limb deficiencies. If you are not an orthopaedic resident, please don't feel unwelcome.

Most orthopaedic surgeons will not be required to look after children with congenital deficiencies of the limbs. These children have such distinctive needs that they are best served by clinics set up specifically for them. However, children everywhere are susceptible to the ravages of trauma, and these children are most likely to come first under the care of general orthopaedic surgeons. Responsible management of these children and their injuries requires an understanding of the differences between these children and adults who are amputees.

With each passing year, the body of specialty medical knowledge grows. It becomes more and more difficult for those responsible for curriculum development to meet the demands of each area of subspecialty interest. We would all like residents to complete their training so fully informed that they know everything possible about each orthopaedic subspecialty. Clearly this is impossible.

How then can we attract the attention of the resident so that OUR area is not forgotten? With that in mind, we have prepared this manual to make the general orthopaedic resident familiar with the principles involved in the care of children with limb deficiencies.

Teaching adults is a challenge far different from that of teaching children. We have borrowed from Dr. Lucy Squires her idea of using short case histories (with appropriate bogus names) to encapsulate and enliven principles with the hope that these principles might be remembered well into the years of orthopaedic practice. We are grateful, too, to Dr. Colin Moseley, from whom we have borrowed the style of "Issues to Ponder."

We would also like you to know about ACPOC, the Association of Children's Prosthetic and Orthotic Clinics. ACPOC was founded on the belief that children with limb deficiencies, whether congenital or acquired through trauma or disease, are best served by specialty clinics in which the combined interest and expertise of a number of people (physicians, be they orthopaedic surgeons, pediatricians or physiatrists; prosthetists; orthotists; physical therapists; occupational therapists; rehabilitation engineers; nurses; psychologists; and social workers) can be brought to bear to help children and their families cope as well as possible with the child's problems.

This is ***not*** meant to be a total guide to prosthetics, but is unabashedly focused on our particular interest—the care of children with limb deficiencies.

Hugh G. Watts, MD
Clinical Professor, Orthopaedics
University of California, Los Angeles
Shriners Hospital for Crippled Children
Los Angeles, California

Mary Williams Clark, MD
Chief, Division of Pediatric Orthopaedics
Department of Orthopaedic Surgery
Medical College of Ohio
Toledo, Ohio

Chapter 1

Test Your Knowledge (Some Illustrative Cases)

The following cases are presented to engender curiosity so that when we come to the "boring" pedantic bits later on, you might stay awake. Also, this section will act as a "pretest" so that you can come back to it later to see how much you learned.

Case # 1
Peter Mowitt

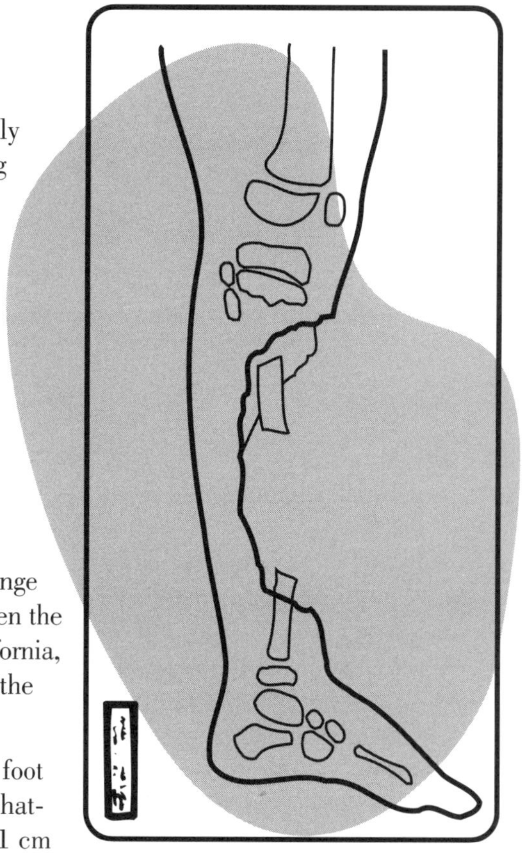

Peter is a 3-year-old boy with a badly traumatized right leg. He was sitting between his father's legs on a power lawnmower. An hour ago, he fell off and the mower ran over his right leg, mangling his foot and ankle and most of his shin. He was brought immediately to you in the emergency room. Keep in mind that all the other orthopaedic surgeons are out of town at the American Academy of Orthopaedic Surgeons (AAOS) annual meeting. You're on your own! (I know it's strange to be mowing grass in February, when the AAOS meets each year, but in California, the grass grows all year, even when the ground shakes.)

None of the tissues of the calf and foot are viable, and the x-rays show a shattered tibia that is broken at about 1 cm below the proximal tibial physis. Several segments of bone are missing.

You advise the parents that Peter's leg needs to be amputated. In spite of an enormous sense of guilt on the father's part, which will probably stay with him for his lifetime and affect all of the subsequent rehabilitation decisions, the family agrees that an amputation is necessary.

You think that there is just enough skin so that you might be able to get closure over the tibial stump. But, split thickness skin grafting over the end of the stump might be required to achieve closure. Because the tibial stump will only be 2 cm long, you realize that Peter will not be able to use a below-knee (BK) prosthesis. In reality, he will function as an above-knee (AK) prosthesis wearer.

Issues to ponder

1. Suppose you think you could barely get closure, giving Peter a *very* short tibial stump. Is it worth it to Peter for you to struggle to keep him as a BK rather than an AK amputee? If so, why? Or should you decide to go for the safer through-the-knee amputation? This will give him an excellent "end-bearing" stump that can be fitted to a "self-suspending" socket because of the flares of the distal femoral condyles.

2. Suppose that the skin loss is so bad that not only can you not do a BK amputation, but you cannot even get enough coverage for a through-knee amputation. Should you go for an AK amputation? What are the consequences for growth? Are there other options?

3. Suppose Peter was 15 years old rather than 3. Would this make a difference in your decision-making?

Comments

1. In general, in an amputation in a child, it is preferable to save as much length as you can. Keep in mind that although he has only 1 cm of bone distal to his proximal tibial physis, that physis has a lot of growing to do. At 3 years of age, a normal boy's tibia would be about 17 cm long, and at maturity it would be about 37 cm long. Between the age of 3 years and maturity, an additional 20 cm of growth will be added to the tibia, and about 55% of this growth will take place in the proximal tibia. This 11 cm of growth plus what he already has could give him a proximal tibial stump of about 12 cm (about 5 inches), which could serve Peter perfectly well as a BK-prosthesis user when he is an adult. In practicality, the tibia may not grow that much because there won't be the same muscle forces applied to the leg, but there is still a very good likelihood that he could be a good BK-prosthesis user.

You are correct that initially, he would indeed have to be fitted with an AK prosthesis and would not be able to control the knee joint. However, gradually, as he got older, he could be converted from an AK to a BK prosthesis user.

In order to save the small amount of below-knee stump, split-thickness skin grafts may certainly be used in a child. Although they would not usually provide adequate coverage for an adult, split-thickness grafts in children usually thicken and can be very useful to save length.

2. If the skin loss is so bad that even the distal femoral physis cannot be saved, this presents major difficulties in ultimate stump length for Peter. At age 3 years, a normal boy's femur would be about 20 cm long. That normal femur would ordinarily grow to about 47 cm (ie, a growth of 27 cm between the ages of 3 years and maturity). However, only a quarter of this growth takes place in the proximal femur (ie, about 6 1/2 cm). Thus, if Peter lost his femur at about 5 cm from his knee joint, he would have an immediate stump length of about 15 cm (6 inches). However, at maturity, his stump would only be about 21 cm (8 ½ to 9 inches) in length, which would be a very short above-knee stump. Clearly then, it would be preferable to save the distal femoral physis if at all possible.

   One thing you could consider is removal of a small segment from the shaft of the femur to allow closure of the skin over the end of the distal femoral epiphysis. This small shortening at the time of his amputation would be more than made up by the 27 cm of growth that could later take place in the distal femur.

   You could also consider leaving the skin open and using skin traction for several days. This can be done with stockinette and tincture of benzoin, gently overwrapped with an elastic bandage. A weight (eg, 1 to 2 kg) is attached to the stockinette and the leg supported in a suspension sling. This may allow a secondary closure.

3. If Peter was 15 years old at the time of the accident and had only a 2-cm proximal tibial stump, the simplest management of his injury probably would be through-knee amputation. However, we want you to keep in mind that as techniques of amputation stump lengthening improve, a small proximal tibial remnant may prove to be useful later.

By the way

Spend some time educating your community that the family lawn mower is a devastatingly efficient amputation machine. Children belong in the house when the lawn is being mowed!

Case # 2
F.I. Bulahgon

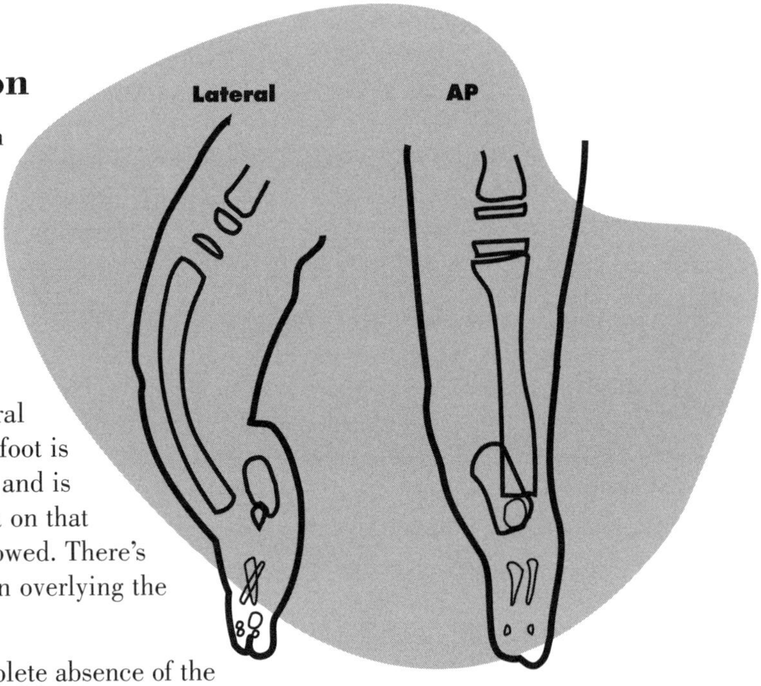

Fred Ivan Bulahgon is a newborn baby who has a deformed foot on the right side. He is otherwise healthy and well. The foot shows an absence of the lateral two rays. The hind foot is in marked equinus and is in valgus. The tibia on that side is short and bowed. There's a dimple in the skin overlying the apex of the bow.

X-rays show a complete absence of the fibula. The tibia has a 30° anterior angulation at midpoint. The foot is missing the lateral two metatarsals, as well as the cuboid. The os calcis and talus are in equinus and marked valgus.

You advise the family that the best management for little Freddie is an operation to remove the deformed foot so that he can be more easily fitted with a prosthesis that would allow him all of the advantages of a full childhood and fulfilled adulthood. The term used by pediatric orthopaedic surgeons to describe such an operation is a "conversion amputation." (Specialists always need special words to make us feel that we are "in the know.")

Issues to ponder

1. Is an amputation the only reasonable option?

2. Is a Syme's amputation the best choice? Your colleague heard that a Boyd amputation would be the best for Freddie. (He's just returned from the AAOS Annual Meeting at which he's learned a lot of new info, and you're not sure what to believe.) What are the pros and cons?

3. Would a BK amputation at midshaft, just above the level of the bow in the tibia, be a reasonable option? What are the pros and cons?

4. What is the best age for Freddie to undergo his amputation?

Comments

1. Is an amputation the only reasonable option? Until now, the answer has been yes. However, as more experience is being gained with correcting the foot deformity by gradual distraction and with anticipation of managing the associated short tibia by lengthening, *some* children with this problem may be managed without an amputation. The problems are prolonged treatment time and the fact that, in spite of all the effort, the child often is left with a deformed and less well functioning foot and ankle.

2. The best level for amputation is a controversial issue. Most orthopaedic surgeons in North America use a Syme's amputation. However, the distal tibia tends to become more penciled, and although it is an end-bearing stump, it may not be as optimal as that seen in a Boyd amputation in which the bulge makes self-suspension easier. By contrast, if the residual tibia is proportionally quite long, the Boyd amputation leaves an unsightly bulge at the ankle level that cannot be masked by the prosthesis. If, however, the tibia is anticipated to be very short so that at maturity the end of the Boyd amputation is at the level of the normal calf, then the bulge can be readily masked within the prosthesis.

   Another option is a "modified Syme's" in which the posterior calcaneal prominence is cut obliquely and left attached to the heel pad. The calcaneal remnant is then fused to the distal tibial *epiphysis,* leaving the physis intact. This procedure can leave a firmer distal stump that is less bulbous, and may endear you to your prosthetist.

3. Would a BK amputation at the midshaft level be a good choice? As a general answer, no. A transdiaphyseal or transmetaphyseal amputation in a child has a moderately high propensity for forming new bone overgrowth at the stump, requiring multiple stump revisions during childhood. Where possible, it is always best to do an amputation that leaves cartilage over the end of the bony stump. The bowing in the tibia is seldom a problem. It usually corrects on its own. Sometimes, it requires later osteotomy to straighten out; however, this is not reason enough to do a midshaft amputation.

4. When is the best age for Freddie to undergo his amputation? In general, you should consider proceeding when a child is starting to pull to a stand. This allows ample time for the child to be old enough to undergo anesthesia safely, for the amputation to heal and the swelling to subside, and for fabrication and fitting of a prosthesis so that all is set when the child is developmentally ready to start walking at about the age of one year.

   A further advantage of amputation at a young age is that the child is less likely to have incorporated the deformed foot into his body image, and an amputation is less likely to be psychologically traumatizing. On the other hand, if the family is not prepared to go ahead with an amputation at that age, it probably is wiser to wait until the parents are ready before proceeding rather than pushing them into a decision that they are unhappy with because of some theoretical psychological reason.

Chapter 2
A Pedantic Overview

Now we get into the boring didactic bits, but who knows, you may remember some of them in years to come.

Most orthopaedic surgeons at some point will have the onerous task of having to do an amputation on a child. If the child is to be well served, the orthopaedist needs to understand the general differences between an adult amputee and a child amputee and, especially, to understand how the growth of the child will impact the management of an amputation. Because the upper extremities are frequently the site of amputations in children, this discussion includes both upper and lower extremities.

"A child is not a small adult" has been the war cry of pediatricians for generations. This certainly is true when it comes to thinking about children with absent limbs, regardless of the cause. In comparison to adult amputees, childhood amputees

- more commonly have congenital limb anomalies;
- more often have the upper extremities involved;
- more often have multiple limbs involved;
- have continually changing developmental capabilities;
- are generally more agile and easier to train to use new devices;
- seldom have associated diseases (such as diabetes) to complicate their care;
- are already dependent persons;
- rarely have serious problems with phantom pain or neuromas;
- have skin that is more tolerant of prosthetic abuse;
- are *not* likely to be careful about the use and maintenance of their prostheses, nor appreciate the costs involved;
- are growing in length and girth;
- have more special needs in prosthetic components; and
- more frequently need to have surgical modifications of their stumps.

These differences are discussed in detail below.

The amputations in children are more commonly congenital than traumatic

Approximately 60% of children seen in amputee clinics have amputations resulting from congenital anomalies. That's what the statistics show. However, many children with traumatic amputations that take place in the community will not end up in the child amputee centers. Traumatic amputations probably are underrepresented in the figures, particularly if they are lower extremity amputations, which are somewhat easier to manage in a less specialized facility. This fact also modifies the next statement.

Children with limb deficiencies more often have the upper extremities involved.

Of children brought to amputee clinics, those with congenital lesions are twice as likely to have the upper extremity involved. Of those children who have acquired amputations, however, only 40% will have the upper extremity involved.

Children with limb deficiencies often have multiple limbs involved.

Approximately 30% of children with congenital limb deficiencies have more than one limb involved (ie, 15% with two limbs, 5% with three limbs, and 10% with all four limbs). By contrast, only 10% of children with traumatic amputations have a loss of more than a single limb.

Wearing a limb prosthesis can be hot, especially in warm climates. Children who have to wear two, or even three or four prostheses, can suffer major problems because there is not enough uncovered skin to lose heat adequately. This problem is greater if the child has a hip or shoulder disarticulation, which requires a prosthesis that covers a considerable area of the trunk. Even reasonable normal activity may be prohibitive in regular weather, let alone in the summer. Such a child understandably may refuse to wear prostheses. In addition, the absence of sensation can be a factor in a child's wish to reject a prosthesis.

The developmental capabilities of children with limb deficiencies or amputations are always changing.

It is obvious that any 2-year-old child is not able to do things that can be done by a 5-year-old child. Nor can the 5-year-old child do the things that a 10-year-old child can do. Children develop appropriate intellectual understanding as well as physical coordination and strength as they grow older. A 1-year-old child who can barely toddle about on two normal legs cannot be expected to manipulate a prosthesis with an articulated knee joint, nor can a 5-year-old child be expected to be able to manage a myoelectrically controlled hand with the same dexterity as a 12-year-old child. Prosthetic components for children need to be appropriate to the developmental age of the child. It is surprising how often this principle is forgotten.

At what age should a child with a lower extremity amputation be fitted? The ideal is to allow the child to stand and walk at the same age as his or her peers. This age would ordinarily be about 1 year. Fitting a child with a lower extremity prosthesis at this age may inhibit the child's ability to crawl, which may be a frustration for the child, but not a major impediment.

If an operation, such as removing a grossly deformed foot, is needed to allow for the proper fit of a prosthesis, at what age should this be done? Surgery should be timed so that there is enough time for the stump swelling to go away and for fabrication of the prosthesis. As a consequence, surgery should be completed when the child is about 9 to 10 months of age.

For a 1-year-old child with an amputation above the knee or at the hip level, the addition of a prosthetic knee joint is not necessary. A 1-year-old child can happily walk with a straight knee, as well as sit with the knee straight because most sitting at this age is done on the floor. The age at which to install a knee joint or to unlock one that is present depends on the child's developmental abilities. This can be done as early as 1.5 to 2 years of age, but there is really very little need to hurry. If a child has any developmental delay, this step can be put off several years without seriously affecting the child's ability to get about.

At what age should a child with an upper extremity amputation be first fitted? Although some have advocated fitting children younger than 6 months of age with upper extremity prostheses so that they can be trained to develop their eye-hand coordination, current practice is to wait until a child is beginning to develop sitting balance, usually at about 5 to 6 months of age. This has been expressed as "Fit with Sit."

At what age should the terminal device in a child's prosthesis be activated? This step also will depend on the child's psychomotor development. Ordinarily, the terminal device is mounted at the time the prosthesis is first applied. At that point, the therapists and parents can open the device and place objects into it so that the child can understand the principle of the device. If a child is to be fitted with a myoelectric prosthesis, some clinics will fit infants very early (at 12 to 24 months) with a simpler single electrode system that alternately controls opening and closing. If a body-powered prosthesis is to be used, the activating cable usually is hooked up at about 1.5 to 2 years of age. Once again, the major factor in the timing of these decisions is the child's developmental readiness.

Children with limb deficiencies or amputations are generally more agile than adults and are easier to train to use new devices.

Children are extremely adaptable. This adaptability makes it easier to manage their lower extremity prosthetics because they will tolerate almost anything that allows them to walk.

Children with multiple limb loss can be extraordinarily adaptable in their abilities to function in the absence of an upper extremity. They readily can be taught to feed themselves and to do many tasks using their feet and toes or to grasp objects between their chin and shoulder or between a very short humeral stump and their chest wall. The sensory feedback that they gain by these maneuvers is an advantage over any prosthesis that we are able to fabricate currently. This ability can cause problems when trying to convince a child to wear an upper extremity prosthesis, because the child may be more facile, certainly initially, without the prosthesis.

In spite of their adaptability, however, children will not tolerate highly technical mechanical devices being applied to them. They usually do so much better without them. This phenomenon is known as ***poor gadget tolerance.*** An almost totally electronic replacement for a deficient upper limb may be an amazement when shown on television, but is rarely accepted by a child.

The increased energy consumption required to propel a prosthesis is not commonly a problem, except in the multilimb deficient child. The recent focus on high technology components for adults has not found a significant place in prosthetics in children.

Although children are ready learners when dealing with a prosthesis, they usually do not share the therapist's enthusiasm for perfection of gait. They usually are quite happy to be able to go from one point to another in their own way. Trying to force them to do otherwise is an exercise in frustration for the therapist and the family. Regardless of what he or she is taught, the child probably will not do it the therapist's way when the adults are not watching. A child may be ready to accept "advanced" gait training in early adolescence when his or her limp may increase with gains in height and weight. This is also a time when the child may become more self-conscious and want to mask the limp if possible.

Children with limb deficiencies or amputations seldom have associated diseases, such as diabetes, to complicate their care.

These children are very likely, however, to have other congenital anomalies that will affect the choice of treatment. (See the next chapter, "Congenital Deficiencies and Their Associated Disorders.")

Children with limb deficiencies or amputations are already dependent persons.

Choosing a treatment plan that requires a long time to complete may not be as much of a problem with a child as it would be with an adult who is employed and may be the family breadwinner. However, the child's dependency increases the number of people who have to be satisfied with the prosthetic management. Not only the patient, but also the parents, and very likely two sets of grandparents as well, will need to be mollified. Children's literature is filled with stories of ugly pirates who have a hook on the end of an amputated arm. What child hasn't heard of Captain Hook and seen vivid pictures that show such people as being evil and fearful? It is not a surprise, therefore, that a child (or the parents) will not be happy with a hook terminal device. The CAPP terminal device does not have that drawback, although a number of parents (but not children) have criticized its appearance as being like that of an alligator. Occasionally it may temporarily be necessary to provide life-like passive hands for an infant in order that a parent will not reject the child.

Although children can be remarkably adaptable, a period of emotional preparation for an amputation will usually be rewarded manyfold with fewer problems. Emotional preparation for amputation needs to include the parents, and often the child's medical caregivers as well, who may become very upset and not deal appropriately with the child.

Children with limb deficiencies or amputations rarely have serious problems with phantom pain or neuromas.

Phantom *sensation* is part of every acquired (but not congenital) amputation. Phantom *pain* (that is, pain that is felt to be in the absent amputated part), however, is usually temporary and rarely a problem. The presence of phantom sensation, while not painful, may be the source of considerable emotional disturbance because the phenomenon is difficult for a child to understand. Preoperative warning and gentle reassurance go much further to solving the problem than medication. Neuromas require surgical care in only about 3% of children.

Children with limb deficiencies or amputations have skin that is more tolerant of prosthetic abuse.

A child's skin is remarkably adaptable. It is not an uncommon sight in underdeveloped countries to see a child with an untreated clubfoot walking on the dorsum of the foot. The skin over the dorsum becomes as thick and callused and capable of full weightbearing as the sole of the foot is in normal children. By the same token, normal skin placed in an end bearing location, if allowed to accept the forces gradually, will readily adapt to weightbearing. In addition, split-thickness skin graft, which in an adult is inappropriate as coverage in the friction areas under a prosthesis, will usually mature and thicken sufficiently in a child. This thickening can allow the orthopaedic surgeon to salvage more distal segments at the time of amputation for acute trauma.

Children with limb deficiencies or amputations are not likely to be careful about the use and maintenance of their prostheses.

Children's components must be durable and safe. A small child is rarely fiscally responsible and does not understand that a myoelectric hand on a forearm prosthesis (costing thousands of dollars) should not be used as a device to hammer on an object. We recall a 10-year-old boy who frequently stabbed a pocket knife through his trouser leg into his AK prosthesis to amaze his friends. Although this allowed him to show them that he really was a "Bionic Man," the socket usually looked as if it had been chewed by a dog.

Durability is an important feature of prosthetic components for children. For example, a SACH (solid ankle cushion heel) foot, while not a component at the forefront of prosthetic technology, is a very reasonable standard for use in a child. When children are older, they may demonstrate a desire for a more responsive foot component; however, the selection of any of the multiple "energy-storing feet" becomes a question of the appropriate use of limited medical resource dollars. Many people in children's limb deficiency clinics are philosophically opposed to this view, and feel that children deserve whatever components will give them the best possible function.

Children outgrow their prostheses in a year or two. Would an average parent provide a $5,000 bike to be used for a year or two for their 7-year-old child, or a Ferrari for their 17-year-old adolescent? However, with a little encouragement from a physician, therapist, or prosthetist, a parent's natural feelings of guilt can lead that parent to spend inordinate amounts on "the latest advance" in prosthetics.

Prosthetic components must allow for the possibility that children may harm themselves or those around them. The metal hook of an upper extremity terminal device can become a dangerous weapon if a small child gets angry and strikes a playmate. Plastic coating to the hook provides a little protection for the playmates as well as for the child's own teeth, were the child to chew on the hook (as any child might be expected to do), but some consider that this plastic coating decreases function.

Children with limb deficiencies or amputations are growing in length and girth.

Children grow. The growth in length is readily attended to by the prosthetist. Sometimes, the need for additional height is overcorrected on the prosthetic side while a small lift is added to the normal side. The lift is easily removed some months later, decreasing the number of times the prosthesis needs to be adjusted. Alternatively, a distal pad can be placed inside the socket and then can be exchanged for a thinner pad with growth.

Children, however, not only grow in length but also in girth. This growth may be sufficiently rapid that if nothing is done to accommodate for it, the need for prosthesis changes will be frequent. Each additional change may mean that the child is without the limb while it is being modified or remade unless there has been good planning for routine maintenance visits. This maintenance time can add up to considerable loss of use. The rapid changes in girth can be accommodated by an expandable socket made out of a lighter weight, more flexible plastic or by having several sleeves, one within the other, that can be progressively discarded as the child grows. Alternatively, the child may initially be fitted with several stump socks that can be removed one by one as needed. However, this may give a sloppy fit at the beginning, and may thus become the source of discomfort as well as skin breakdown.

Children with limb deficiencies or amputations have more special needs in prosthetic components.

The first obvious need is that of small size. This refers not only to the overall dimensions but also to the weight. In general, prosthetic components for adults come in large, medium, and small sizes, with perhaps an extra small for women. Obviously, children need an array of sizes that range from what may be fitted to a tiny 1-year-old child up to that needed by a teenager of the smallest adult proportions. At this point, the economic factor becomes operative. Manufacturers of prosthetic components cannot reasonably be expected to fabricate and store large stocks of multiple-sized items that have a low turnover.

Weight becomes a particular problem, not only because of the smaller muscle mass available to move prosthetic components but also because children with multiple limb involvement find that minor difficulties with a component involving one limb may adversely affect the functioning of another limb.

Children with multiple limb involvement frequently require considerable individualization of components. This typically requires custom fabrication. For example, an 8-year-old boy who was born with bilateral hip disarticulations and an absent hand on the left, was able to walk on bilateral lower extremity prostheses by using a regular forearm crutch under his normal right arm and by having a specially made crutch built as the terminal device of the left upper extremity prosthesis. In order that he could be functional when he wasn't walking, the left upper extremity prosthesis was fitted with a quick-disconnect wrist joint at which he could easily exchange the crutch for a hook terminal device. Fabrication of such special items is costly and can present many difficulties in finding funding for these children. At the same time, it provides the stimulus to creativity to those dealing with such children.

Children with limb deficiencies or amputations more frequently need to have surgical modifications of their stumps.

Children with congenital deletions will often have sufficient deformity of the extremity stumps that fitting with prostheses becomes a challenge. In such children, it is often preferable to modify the deformity surgically by either removing a segment that is in the way or straightening it in order to allow for better fitting. Such a procedure is usually called a "conversion amputation."

Improving a stump to provide better function may include fusion of several limb segments. This fusion allows the retention of length and gives a single rigid lever with which the child can propel the prosthesis. This fusion characteristically is done in children with PFFD (proximal femoral focal deficiency), in which the very short femoral segment is fused to the tibia. If necessary, it can be done at the level of the bony secondary centers of ossification, thereby permitting continued growth at one or both physes. This procedure not only provides a better single segment stump, it also brings the line of weightbearing closer to the center of gravity of the body, resulting in much more functional prosthetic wearing.

Much has been written about the preference for doing "conversion amputations" before the age of about 1 year, when a child is less likely to miss the part removed. However, when the child is at that age, it is often very difficult for parents to accept the need to remove parts. They may well harbor an underlying hope that somewhere there exists someone who can correct the deformity, thereby avoiding the need for amputation. If that is the case, children appear to be sufficiently adaptable in their psychic needs that a delay in doing a "conversion amputation" for several years until the parents are comfortable with the idea is not a major problem for the child. However, 2 years of age is a bad time at which to do an elective amputation. Mind you, 2 years of age (the "NO!" year) is a bad time to try most anything.

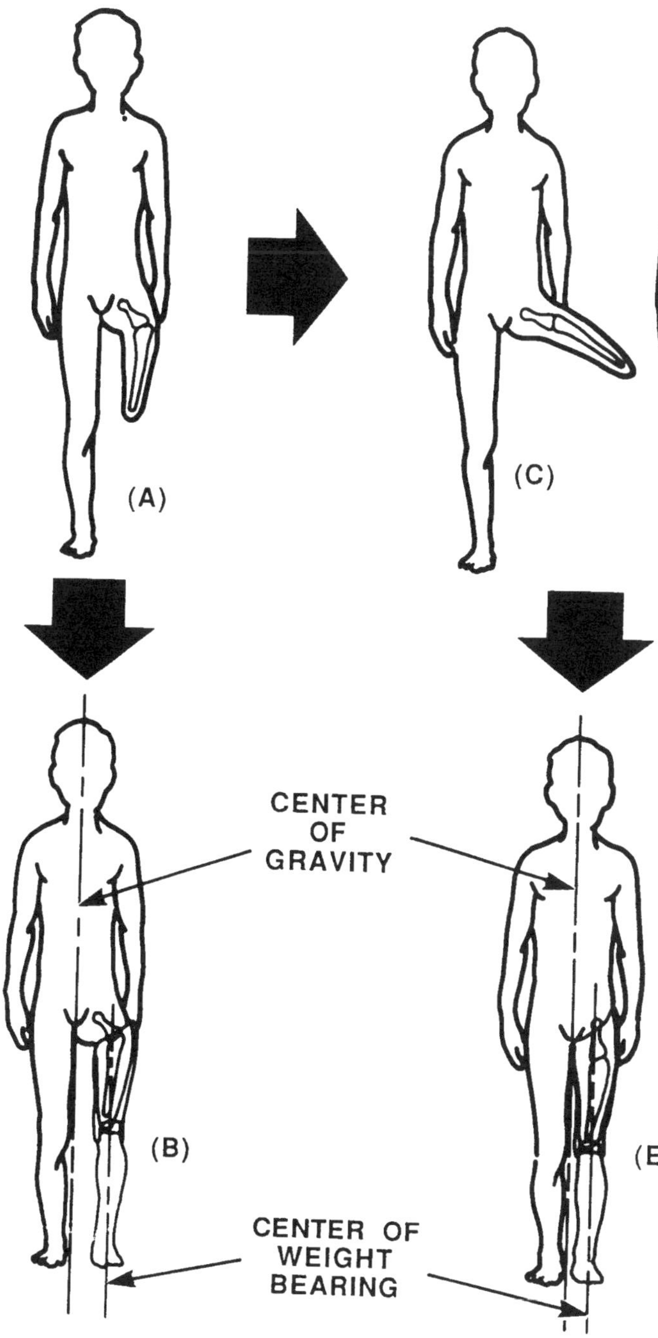
(A)
(C)
(D)
CENTER
OF
GRAVITY
(B)
(E)
CENTER OF
WEIGHT
BEARING

Chapter 2

The Impact of Skeletal Growth and Remodeling on Amputations in Children

There are two special issues that must be kept in mind when doing amputations in children: (1) growth and remodeling of the skeleton and (2) the propensity of children to develop "overgrowth," which greatly hampers their function, at the end of their amputated bones.

Growth and Remodeling of the Skeleton

Growth in length can be an important issue. If a child requires an amputation through the diaphysis of the femur, for example, the growth in the distal femur is lost (representing 75% of the growth for that bone). What began as a long AK stump at the time of amputation in an infant ends up as a very short AK stump by the time that child becomes an adult. Consequently, it is fundamentally important that all epiphyses be saved if possible. If skin closure is a problem, try split-thickness skin grafts, or consider shortening the bone by taking a segment out of the diaphyseal area to allow the distal segment to move proximally so that the skin may be brought around the end of the stump.

Remodeling of bones, such as straightening a bowed tibia in a child with a congenital deletion of the fibula, can be advantageous. But remodeling can also create problems. In adults, a right-angle osteotomy of the distal humerus can be done to provide rotational control for patients with above elbow amputations. This allows them to reach over their heads while wearing their prostheses without the prosthesis spinning on the stump. If such an operation is done in a child, the bone will gradually straighten out to negate the beneficial effects of the osteotomy.

Terminal Overgrowth

Overgrowth of amputation stumps in children has always been a problem and can even occur in congenital amputees. It particularly is a problem in the humerus, the fibula, and the tibia. About 15% of juvenile patients who have amputations before the age of 12 years require revision, whereas while this does not happen if the amputation is done at a later age. Yet, if children required stump revisions previously and they are now older than 12 years of age, overgrowth could occur repeatedly. It has been well documented that this overgrowth is not a result of stimulation of the physis proximally but of the development of appositional new bone on the end of the stump.

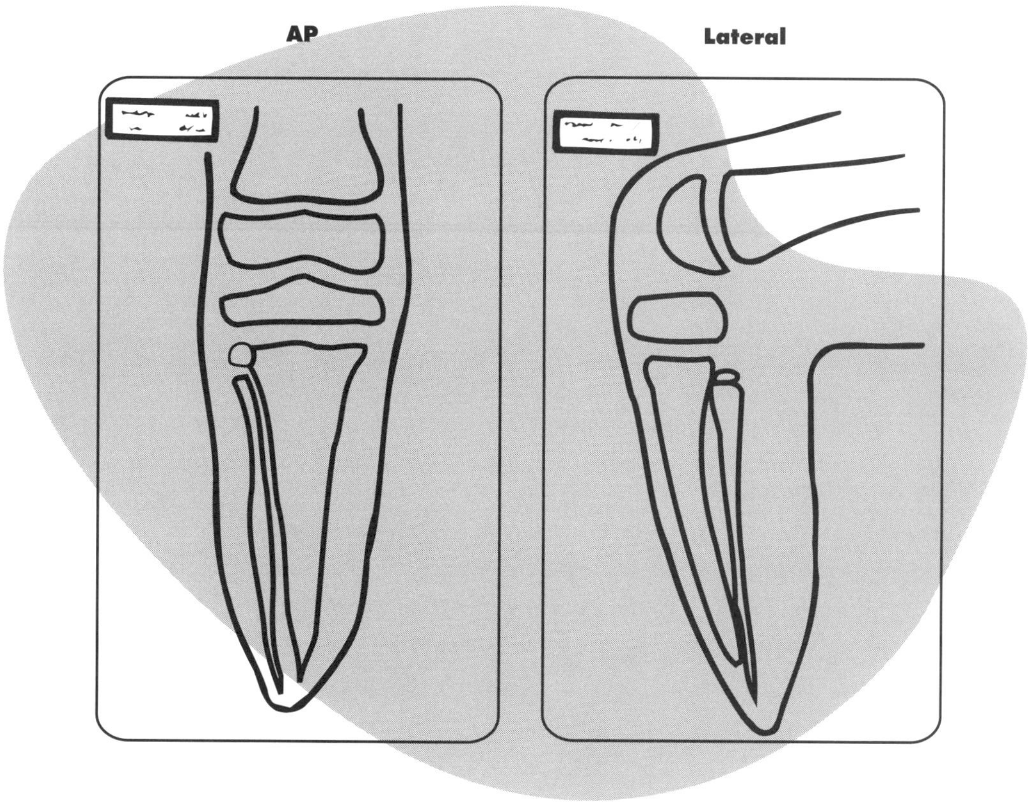

The easiest way to manage the problem is to avoid it by performing amputations, where possible, through a joint so that the end of the bone is covered by its normal cartilage. If this is not possible, a number of maneuvers have been used with varying success.

In children who have had amputations for tumors and then receive postoperative chemotherapy, overgrowth at the end of an amputation stump must be differentiated from soft-tissue retraction. In such children, the chemotherapy adversely influences the healing of the fascia so that the muscles draw proximally, leaving the bone protruding subcutaneously. If a stump revision is done while the child is still receiving chemotherapy, the process is likely to be repeated soon thereafter. Several revisions may lead to an unfortunately short stump. It is better, if possible, to wait until 3 to 6 months after the cessation of the chemotherapy to do a definitive procedure.

Chapter 3

What Have You Learned? (Congenital Deficiencies and Their Associated Disorders)

It's strange how this is the kind of stuff that shows up on In-Service examinations.

(Of course, YOU don't need to worry)

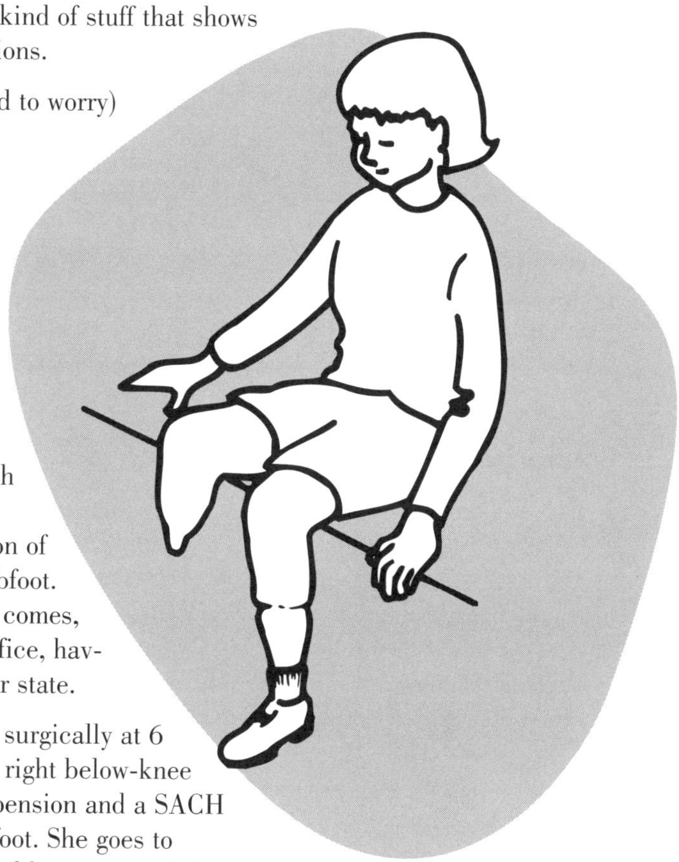

Case #3
A.M. "Neon" Bands

Alice Marie is known as "Neon" to her family because they think of her as such a bright and bubbly child. She was born with several missing fingers, an open below-knee amputation of the right leg, and a left clubfoot. She is now 4 years old and comes, with her parents, to your office, having just moved from another state.

Her clubfoot was corrected surgically at 6 months of age. She wears a right below-knee prosthesis, with sleeve suspension and a SACH (solid ankle cushion heel) foot. She goes to preschool, is very active, and keeps up with her peers. They have come to see you for two reasons.

Neon was this couple's first child. Initially stunned by her differences, they determined not to have more children. However, they now see her as the charming normal child she is, and they are feeling that they would like her to have a sibling after all. They ask, "Should we risk having another child of our own, or should we adopt a child?"

Neon has recently begun complaining at the end of the day that her leg hurts. She has had scabs at the end of the leg. When she picks at the scabs, they drain. The parents leave the prosthesis off a few days (Neon's an accomplished and independent "hopper"), the open area heals, and then the process repeats itself in a week or so.

Issues to Ponder

1. Can you determine the etiology of her congenital differences by history alone? (How about an educated guess?)

2. What examination findings might help you?

3. Does she need a chromosome analysis? (Do her parents?)

4. What do you tell her parents about their family planning?

5. What is the likely etiology of the skin problem on her residual limb (stump)?

6. What other congenital limb deficiency may be acquired in utero? Here's a hint: The preponderance of congenital below-elbow limb deletions occur on the left side.

Comments

1. The history of an "open" below-knee amputation at birth suggests strongly that Neon has had amniotic bands ("constriction bands") in utero; the clubfoot is also suggestive evidence. There is an increased incidence of clubfoot in congenital constriction band syndrome, which we used to call "Streeter's dysplasia." The increased incidence of clubfoot is thought to be secondary to the oligohydramnios that is a result of the loss of fluid through the amniotic tear, which also produces the bands that wrap around the limbs.

2. A full or partial ring or band on a finger or other limb part would be confirmatory. (The missing fingers and transverse deficiency of the leg could be developmental, and the open BK amputation could be an erroneous history, or a forceps or episiotomy (!) injury. Stranger things have happened.)

3. No, Neon does not need to have chromosome analysis done, nor do her parents. There are no reports of familial congenital bands. Their risk of having another affected child equals that of the general population, which is at least 1 in 5,000.

4. It is extremely unlikely that they would have another child with constriction band syndrome. (Never say never. We don't know what factors contribute to the amniotic rupture that starts the band sequence, and another child with band syndrome may not have such an easy time of it. The bands can be swallowed by the fetus and cause midface clefting or can wrap around the head and cause hydrocephalus. The developing fetal ectoderm can contact the 'bare' chorion and adhere, causing omphalocele, bladder extrophy, or other deformities.)

5. The current problem with pain and recurrent breakdown at the end of her stump may be due to distal overgrowth of the tibia or fibula. (See Case #5, pp 24-28.) After you examine her, you should take x-rays of the stump, AP and lateral, to examine the state of the bone there. A tapered bone end is "overgrowth." Prosthetic modification may improve symptoms for a while, but most children will need some surgical revision. (*See* Case #7, pp 31-32)

   It is particularly important to remember that Neon has a limb deficiency that was acquired in utero. It is not a genetic defect, but a mechanical mishap. The amnion, inner layer of the membranes surrounding the fetus, tears, and the strands of amnion become wrapped around the waving parts of the fetus, usually arms or legs. Because these amniotic bands will not expand, they cause constriction and vascular compromise as the part grows.

6. Very possibly, the most common congenital limb deficiency of all, the below-elbow deletion, may be an acquired intrauterine amputation. This deletion, known in international terminology as a transverse deficiency of the forearm, (usually) occurs in its proximal one third. No one knows why this is the most common deletion. It certainly is a curious observation. Some believe the etiology may be thrombi in the placenta, which loosen and embolize, via the fetal circulation, to the brachial artery bifurcation. This etiology would explain the significant (3:1) predominance of left-sided lesions, because of streaming and flow characteristics, and the less sharp curve of the aorta to the left (rather than right) subclavian. What is the chance of recurrence of such a deficiency in the same family? It is negligible. We could legitimately call it a "congenital amputation," because it is not a developmental defect.

Case #4
Radia L. deFissionsea

Radia Louise is a newborn baby, whom you are called to see in the nursery because of her right hand deformity. She has only three fingers, without an apparent thumb, and the hand deviates significantly "inward" (away from the distal ulna). The distal ulna is easily palpable. You can only feel one very short forearm bone. When you check the elbow you can passively flex and extend it, and you see Radia actively flexing it. But you are not sure about extension. Is it only gravity? She also moves the hand a bit.

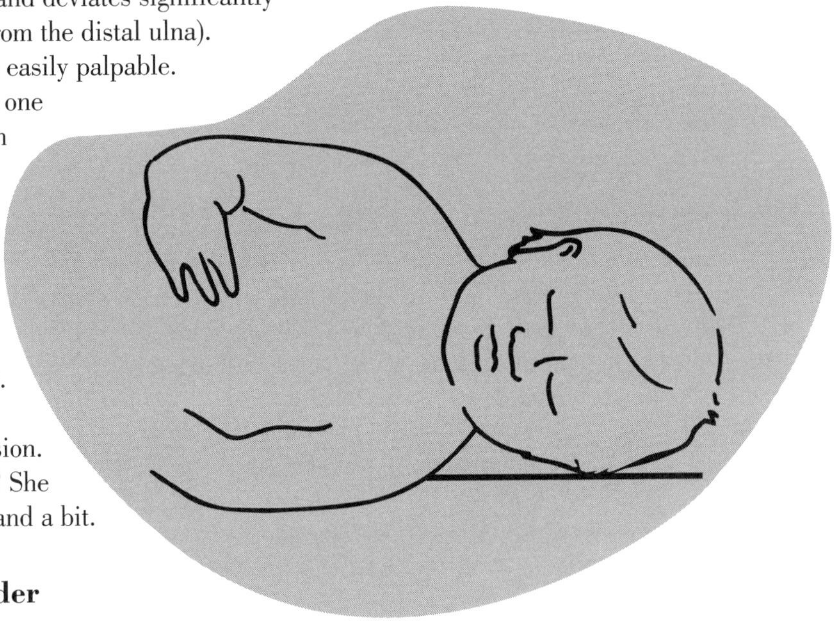

Issues to ponder

1. Before you see the x-ray, what do you expect to see?

2. What further examination of Radia, beyond the right arm, should you do? What tests, if any, would you suggest ordering?

Comments

1. You will probably see a single bone in the forearm, with its proximal end resembling an ulna. In the hand, there will probably be three full rays (metacarpals and all associated phalanges). At least that is what you expect, but there may be all sorts of variations.

2. You want to be sure to do a complete examination. Start with the appendage most orthopaedists only glance at, the head. Check the cranial nerves (remember those eponyms?), especially VII; check the palates (soft and hard); check the eyes and ears for placement and formation. Work downward, not neglecting the chest. Check for proper number and placement of nipples, and check the pectoral muscles. Is there a heart murmur? Check the bottom of the baby. Does she have a normal anus? And, do the rest of the usual orthopaedic examination. Carefully check the other extremities for even minor abnormalities, which could make this child's diagnostic (and possibly prognostic) category change from a single-limb problem to a multilimb problem (eg, hypoplastic thumb, extra-wide, possibly duplicate syndactilized toes, and so forth). Are there petechiae or bruises that might suggest TAR (thrombocytopenia with absent radius) syndrome? Ask the mother and the nurses in the newborn nursery about the child's sucking and swallowing. (Could there be tracheolaryngeal abnormalities?) Is the child urinating normally? (Might there be renal anomalies?)

What tests should you order? Probably all children in this category (radial limb deficiency) should have complete and differential blood cell counts *and* a platelet count, a renal ultrasound, and a chest x-ray to evaluate the heart.

Why all the fuss? There are at least 21 named syndromes that have radial deficiency associated with them, and you may be the first to alert the rest of the baby's medical team to occult and potentially life-threatening abnormalities. (There is a good discussion of this issue in a whole chapter in Michael Goldberg's book, *The Dysmorphic Child: An Orthopedic Perspective,* Raven Press, 1987.) There are two syndromes that you should be on the alert for.

In the first, the child has Radia's problem as well as an anal atresia; although the urine is normal, an ultrasound shows abnormal kidney collecting systems and hydroureter. The chest film shows a normal heart but two block vertebrae in the lumbar spine. This is young **Vladimir Alfred Terre,** who has VATER association: Vertebral/ventricular, Anal, Tracheo-Esophageal, Radial/renal problems. (VATER is really easier than VVATERR to remember.)

In the second syndrome, the child has bilaterally symmetric radial absences and very short humeri, with all rays present on the hands (but stiff interphalangeal joints and hypoplastic thumbs). When you see him in the newborn nursery, he also has some bruising. This is **Thaddeus Acrucius Roadpaver,** who has TAR syndrome. He needs immediate complete blood cell and platelet counts! The thrombocytopenia part of TAR (thrombocytopenia with absent radius) syndrome may produce damaging bleeding (even death) if platelets are not given in the first several days of life. His middle name, Acrucius, is to remind you to check the knees. The more severely involved children with TAR syndrome have dysplastic or missing knee ligaments (or even have fusion between the femur and tibia or, more properly, nonsegmentation). The key to recognizing children with TAR syndrome in the nursery is the symmetry and the presence of all digits in spite of the absent radii.

Now that you have had a chance to read through the details, try your hand at the next cases (as a posttest, if you will) to see what you remember.

Case #5
Paul Frederick Foster Dietz IV

Paul is 2 weeks old and was born with a very short left leg. The pediatrician in the newborn nursery had taken an x-ray that showed the left tibia to be about the same length as the one on the right, but the femur is missing its upper parts and is less than half the length of the femur on the right.

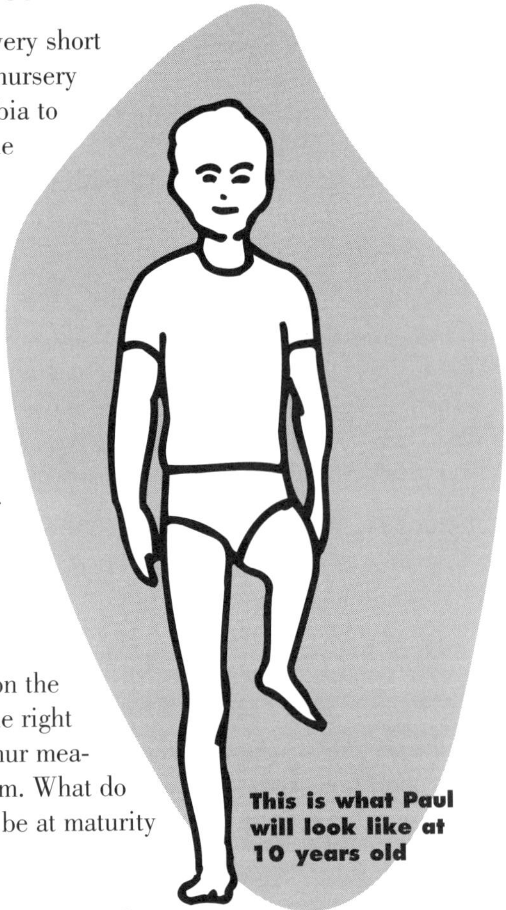

Issues to ponder

1. What is Paul's diagnosis?

2. Paul's parents ask you "How long will his left leg be when he finishes growing? Can you tell us now how much of a difference there will be between the lengths of his two legs when he's grown up?"

   You measure the lengths of the bones on the x-ray taken in the newborn nursery. The right femur measures 10 cm and the left femur measures 4 cm. The tibias are equal at 7 cm. What do you expect his leg length difference to be at maturity if nothing is done?

3. Your colleague looks at the x-ray and points out that, because of the hip flexion contracture, the AP view of the left femur is really a flexed view looking obliquely down the shaft, and the measurement that you got is really not accurate. You request a lateral x-ray of both femurs and find that

the right femur measures 10 cm and the left measures 6 cm. Does this change the outlook for Paul? What new options do you want to consider?

4. Paul's left foot is quite deformed. He is missing the lateral three rays, and it looks as if the bones of the hind foot are deformed. Does this alter your options for Paul?

Comments

1. Paul has a PFFD, a proximal femoral focal deficiency. In spite of its name, the problems are not focal in the proximal femur. The distal femur is usually dysplastic, and there is considerable anterior-posterior ligamentous laxity, which can be a source of problems if femoral lengthening is to be considered. Furthermore, the acetabulum is commonly involved (sometimes to the extent that it is virtually nonexistent) and the proximal musculature around the hip is not usually normal, so even if there is a stable hip joint, there may be an abductor limp.

2. Paul's parents have asked you what is going to happen in the future. How can you make an educated guess? As a general rule, the principle of "proportionality in growth" is a very useful first approximation. The x-ray that you have from the newborn nursery is not an orthoroentgenogram or a scanogram; however, the body parts are so small that there is relatively little magnification in the x-ray. With that in mind, you can measure the length of the different bones on the x-ray and have reasonable approximation of the actual bone lengths.

   In children with congenital deformities, usually the deficient part grows proportionally with the normal side. For example, if the short femur is currently at 50% of the normal femur, it can reasonably be assumed that at maturity, the short femur will be 50% of the normal femur's length. In this case the right femur measured 10 cm and the left measured 4 cm (40% of the opposite side). A normal male femur at maturity is approximately 47 cm in length; therefore, the short femur can be expected to grow to about 19 cm, giving an ultimate shortness on the left femur of 28 cm. This then gives you something to work with in making long-run plans. It is important to stress to the parents that this is only a first approximation, and as the child grows and some more x-rays are obtained, the number can be refined.

3. It is certainly important that the x-rays you use to obtain your measurements are properly taken. The shorter the femoral segment, the more likely it is that the child will hold the femur flexed and the harder it is to take a true AP x-ray. Lateral views are a useful way of getting better measurement films.

Certainly if the short femur now measures 0.6 of the long femur, then the anticipated left femoral length at maturity would be about 28 cm, and the leg-length discrepancy anticipated at maturity about 19 cm. Although this is a great deal, it does start to put Paul into the category of potential femoral lengthening at a later date. It is not necessary to anticipate lengthening the full amount of the discrepancy. Combining an epiphysiodesis (say for 5 cm), wearing an inside heel lift of 1.5 cm, and leaving the leg about 2 cm short reduces the femoral lengthening problem to about 10 cm, which is within the limits of consideration.

4. A van Nes rotationplasty is a consideration in treating children with PFFD. In this procedure, the leg is rotated 180°, the ankle joint is used as a controllable knee joint, and a below-knee-type prosthesis can be applied to the foot, converting what would have been an above-knee situation to a below-knee situation. However, if Paul's foot is deformed (parts are missing and the ankle and subtalar joints do not move well), a van Nes procedure clearly is not indicated.

More issues to ponder

5. Suppose that Paul was 4 years old when you first saw him. His right femur measures 25 cm and the left measures 7 cm, the right tibia measures 19 cm and the left measures 18 cm. The foot is deformed, and he has little motion in the ankle or subtalar joints. Another doctor has advised the family that the most propitious way for Paul to lead an effective childhood, and in the long-run a most effective adulthood, would be for Paul to undergo a Syme's amputation of the foot and be fitted as an above-knee prosthesis wearer.

   Do you agree? What are the alternatives? The family agree and Paul has the surgery recommended and is well fitted as an above-knee prosthesis wearer.

6. One year later, when you see Paul you note that his prosthesis stands out lateral from his normal leg. You reason, correctly, that this is because of his very proximal flexed knee. You propose to the family that you fuse Paul's knee. What are the possible advantages of a fused knee?

7. You recognize that his above-knee stump may now end up too long at maturity. Why is that?

8. To manage the problem of a too-long thigh stump at maturity, you propose to alter the lengths at the time that you do the knee fusion. Are you going to leave both the distal femoral and the proximal tibial physes, cut away his distal femoral physis, cut away his proximal tibial physis, or do you cut away both? How do you decide?

9. Suppose that Paul was a bit different when you saw him. Now, he has a normal foot and ankle with normal motor power. What else can you consider?

More comments

5. The other doctor has given sound advice to the family. With his short femur measuring only 7/25ths of the normal side, he will have a 34-cm leg-length discrepancy from the femurs and approximately another 2-cm shortness from the tibias. This is clearly outside the possibility of lengthening. With his deformed foot and ankle, a van Nes rotationplasty is not indicated. An amputation of the deformed foot so that he can be properly fitted with an above-knee prosthesis is the desirable way to go. The removal of the foot may be done as a Syme's amputation or, possibly, as a Boyd amputation, depending on the anatomy of the residual foot (see Freddie's case #2, page 4).

6. The patient's own anatomic knee joint, which really is functioning at the level of the high thigh on the opposite side, creates an extra link in the thigh segment of the patient's stump. This extra link makes it more difficult for Paul to control his prosthesis. Furthermore, there is a great tendency for the knee to be kept flexed and the back of the thigh, on the short side, used to sit on the rim of the prosthetic socket. This situation places the whole prosthesis more laterally than on the normal side and means that in midstance, Paul has to lean considerably further to the left to get his weight over his foot (see figure on page 24). This aggravates the propensity for an abductor lurch caused by weakness of the abductor muscles, which is part of this disease, and/or by the instability of the hip joint. By fusing the tibia to the femur (*in the line of the femur*), the whole segment is brought down parallel to the opposite thigh, and now the prosthetic foot can be placed closer to the midline.

7. How long should the thigh segment be on the Syme's amputation side? Paul is now 5 years old, and his right normal femur is approximately 26 cm in length. When he reaches skeletal maturity, it will be 47 cm in length. At skeletal maturity, the end of the left stump needs to be short enough above his normal knee to allow for a prosthetic knee joint to be built in at the same level as his normal knee. Keep in mind that in addition to the end of his bony stump (ie, the distal tibia), there will be about 1 to 2 cm of soft tissue and then a socket that needs to be attached to the metal knee joint. Thus, a difference of 10 cm (between the bone ends) would be ideal. Although this difference can be less (by using more expensive special knee joints or by leaving him with different knee heights), it would be preferable if the end of his tibia was at 37 cm at maturity. However, at the present time, his left tibia alone measures 18 cm and will grow to approxi-

mately 37 cm itself. To that must be added his 7 cm of present femur and the 6 cm (7/25 x (47-25)) that his short femur will grow. If everything is left intact, his left thigh stump will measure 50 cm, which is 13 cm too long!

8. To manage the problem of a too-long thigh stump at maturity, a little simple mathematics can give you an estimate of what needs to be left, if anything, in the way of distal femoral and proximal tibial physis. Keep in mind that the tibia grows in its distal end at approximately one half the rate of the opposite normal distal femur, so his short stump will need to start out too long to allow the normal femur to catch up then overtake the opposite abnormal leg.

9. If Paul had a normal foot and ankle with normal motor power of the joints, he could be considered for a van Nes rotationplasty. When should this be done? Characteristically, children who have their rotationplasties done as small children tend to derotate and require a repeat rotation. Newer techniques include detaching quadriceps and hamstrings distally before rotation, then reattaching (hamstrings to gastronemii, quadriceps and adductors to anterior and lateral compartment fascia). This decreases the incidence of derotation. Other options are to wait until the child is older than 10 years of age and do a definitive procedure versus doing the procedure at a much younger age and allowing the child the benefits of the van Nes procedure in the anticipation that a repeat rotationplasty will be needed a number of years later. That decision needs to be made in consultation with the parents. Keep in mind that at maturity, you would want the short leg to have the ankle/knee ("kankle") at the level of the normal knee at maturity. The point of ankle motion is best estimated as being at the tip of the fibular malleolus. Knee fusions are just as appropriate in children undergoing van Nes rotationplasties as in those having a Syme's procedure, and the appropriate length can be managed as discussed above.

Case #6
Amelia Armor

Amelia is a 1-year-old girl who was born without arms. She has small residual scapulae that she is able to shrug with. She is intelligent and very cooperative.

The week before Amelia came to see you in the office, you had heard a lecture on prosthetics in children and learned that children missing parts of upper extremities were usually first fitted with prostheses when they were able to sit independently (which Amelia is currently able to do easily). Feeling confident that you have heard the latest information on the subject, you tell the family that Amelia is now old enough to be fitted for upper extremity prostheses and refer her to the local Children's Amputee Clinic. The parents are overjoyed that something is finally being done for their little girl.

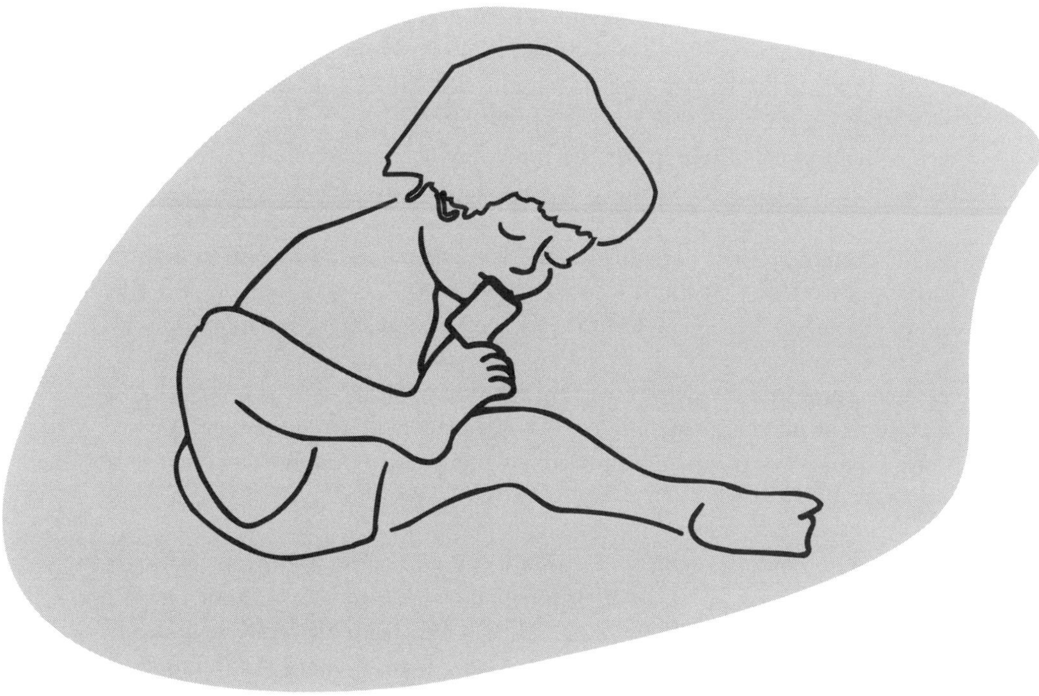

Issues to ponder

1. What kind of prosthesis do you think this child will use when she is mature?
2. With this in mind, what sort of prosthesis do you think that you would order for her at this time?
3. When you saw her in your office, you forgot to examine her feet, knees, and hips. Why is this evaluation important in planning Amelia's management?
4. What else is easy to overlook?
5. What role do you think an occupational therapist could play in this child's care?
6. Are there any associated disorders that you would want to warn the parents about?

Comments

1. Most children who are born with the absence of both arms will not wear prostheses during their lifetime. In spite of all the developments in the field of modern prosthetics, the lack of proprioception, the weight, and the discomfort of heat retention are such that children find that they can do much better on their own without prosthetic help. By the time they reach adulthood, they are able to do almost everything for themselves with their feet.

   It is important to keep in mind that these comments relate to children born without arms. Older children who lose their arms due to trauma are much more likely to struggle to replace what they have become accustomed to.

   At some point in their lives, especially during adolescence, some children born without arms may request simple cosmetic arms to be used for special occasions. (Remember that children born without arms are not born without normal hormones.)

2. With this in mind, common sense would lead you not to prescribe any prosthesis. However, there are many other forces that come to bear. Initially, most parents are desperate to try to fit such a child with prosthetic arms. As a consequence, a trial of prosthetic fitting may be a necessary stage that a family must go through so that they can experience, personally, the rejection of the prostheses by the child. With this in mind, the prescription of a set of arm prostheses with expensive myoelectric components is not a practical way to proceed.

3. Because Amelia probably will not use prosthetic arms and will function by using her feet in place of her hands, it is important to know the status of her motion and muscle control of her hips, knees, ankles, and toes. Because one congenital anomaly is so frequently accompanied by a number of others, the absence of arms makes it reasonably possible that there may be missing or deformed parts of the lower extremity.

4. "One congenital anomaly is frequently accompanied by a number of other anomalies" does not refer only to the musculoskeletal system. Remember that 4 to 7 weeks of gestation is the same time during which other organs are forming as well as the limbs. So think especially about the kidneys and heart.

5. Although the occupational therapist's skills in prosthetic training will probably play a very limited part in Amelia's care, because in the long run she will not wear protheses, an occupational therapist will be of fundamental importance in teaching Amelia how best to substitute her missing arms with her feet.

Furthermore, the ability to shrug her shoulders can be very useful to her for grasping objects between the side of her neck and her shoulder. The use of assistive devices (eg, a mouth stick for typing when she gets older) can help Amelia deal with the world. Toileting is one of the major problems that a child without arms has difficulties with.

6. These children have an increased chance of developing scoliosis (not of the congenital variety). If the scoliosis should become evident, the curves are notoriously resistant to bracing. But, if you consider a spine fusion, ponder at length what might happen to the child's ability to reach the mouth with the feet. Weigh the advantages and disadvantages of the child's lifetime functions, not the x-rays.

Case #7
Capistrano de Bono

Capistrano, known to his school chums as "Cap," is 11 years old. Five years ago, he was playing on his older brother's three-wheeled All Terrain Vehicle. He made too sharp a turn, and the vehicle rolled over on top of him, crushing his left leg at midtibia. His brother saw the accident, shouted to his father who ran out to the boy. The father and the older brother were able to turn the vehicle upright and extricate Cap and rush him to the hospital in the family's pick-up.

In the 5 years since Cap had his accident, he has been remarkably functional in his below-knee prosthesis; he is able to go to school, to play baseball, and even to play football.

He has a problem now. He is getting a sore at the end of his stump. It is the second time this has happened. The last time, 3 years ago, he had to have an operation in which the end of his tibia was trimmed back. He could not go to school for a week and lost 4 weeks of wearing his prosthesis until the swelling went down, and the new socket could be made for him. That cost him the season on the Little League team. It was a very long month for Cap. (*See* Case #3 figure, p 19)

Issues to ponder

1. What's likely to happen to Cap next?

2. What might have been done when he was first seen in the hospital 5 years ago that might have decreased Cap's difficulties?

3. What do you propose to do now?

Comments

1. Once a child demonstrates that he/she will develop terminal overgrowth, the probability is very high that the problem will recur every 2 to 4 years. An x-ray at this time will show the end of his tibia/fibula to have a sharp tapered spike that may eventually protrude through the skin if nothing is done.

2. Children who undergo amputations across the shaft of the bones have a great tendency to develop terminal overgrowth, especially if the amputation takes place in a child younger than 11 years of age.

   Knowing this, the surgeon could have used a piece of Cap's metatarsal head (or some other salvageable piece of bone with a cartilage cap) at the original operation. If the piece being salvaged might be infected, common sense would lead you not to use it. But remember, the cartilage-capped piece of bone does not have to be living.

3. Because Cap has demonstrated that he probably is a candidate for frequent stump revisions, and bone trimming is unlikely to be a satisfactory procedure for him at this time, consider capping the end of the tibia with something. Silastic caps have not done well. Stainless steel caps have been equally disappointing. Try a biologic cap. The proximal fibula works well. (Besides, you can remove all of the fibula so it won't develop terminal overgrowth, but if so, excise it extraperiostially). Some surgeons prefer to use iliac apophyseal cartilage (an obvious choice if there is no proximal fibula).

By the way

Three-wheeled ATVs are very dangerous (because of their instability during turns). Are they still legal in your state? Do some preventive politicking!

Case #8
Myra Olivia Lectra

Myra is 7 years old. She was born with the distal half of her left forearm missing. (Our jargon would classify her as "a congenital BE," an obviously dehumanizing term meaning below-elbow limb deficiency.)

Myra got along pretty well with her stump. She could do most everything. She liked to help her mom in the kitchen. Making sandwiches was a favorite, and she loved to ladle on the mayonnaise, so she got the nickname Myo.

Her parents saw a television program, "That's Incredible," that showed a man with a bionic arm, so they took her to the big city amputee clinic so she could be fitted with one of the same things.

Issues to ponder

1. What are the advantages to fitting Myo with a myoelectric prosthesis?
2. What might be the disadvantages?
3. The parents have seen a myoelectrically controlled arm on the television. They may see other children with similar prostheses at the clinic. If Myo gets fitted with one, will her parents be happy with how it looks and works?
4. Suppose Myo's father is extremely wealthy? What difference would this make?

Comments

1. A myoelectric prosthesis does not need an extensive harness to keep it on. Typically, the supracondylar socket design provides adequate suspension. These prostheses are usually quite cosmetic.
2. Myoelectric prostheses are expensive. A standard myoelectric below-elbow prosthesis might cost $8,000. They also are more likely to break down and, of course, the batteries may fail. If a child lives some distance from the prosthetic facility, the repair turnaround time may not be practical.
3. Even when shown what one looks like, that final production is almost always a disappointment, at least initially. It just is not a real arm, which is what most parents are secretly wishing for.
4. The financial support makes it much more likely that repairs will not be a problem for Myo. The family can have two complete units, so that one is always available in event of a breakdown. However, people accustomed to being able to buy anything they want may be more disappointed that their daughter cannot be given a real arm.

Case #9
Purpurina Fulminans

Purpurina was 5 years old when she caught the chicken pox that all the kids in the neighborhood were sharing. However, she had an unusual complication with disseminated intravascular clotting. This led to gangrenous loss of the tip of her nose, all the fingers of her left hand at the proximal interphalangeal joints, her right thumb totally, and part of each leg—the right below the knee, and the left at the level of the knee joint.

In spite of this devastating problem, Purpurina is a cheerful, bright teenager who always charms those whom she meets. She wears a right below-knee prosthesis and a left knee disarticulation prosthesis. She is happy with her hand function and doesn't feel that she needs anything done for her hands.

Issues to ponder

1. What other diseases can result in similar disseminated clotting with loss of extremities?

2. Purpurina used to enjoy swimming. When she was 8 years old, she wanted to try swimming again, but her parents worried that it would not be safe for her to swim. What would you have advised her parents?

3. Now she is in high school, and her classmates are going on a ski trip. Purpurina wants to go with them and ski. Is that realistic?

Comments

1. The condition, commonly known as purpura fulminans, can follow infections with meningococcemia or other bacteria, eg, pneumococci.

2. Swimming is a good sport for amputees and can be readily done by those with no legs whatsoever.

3. Sure it is, but she will need help. She will need to modify her right below-knee prosthesis (or even have a separate ski leg made) to allow her foot to be dorsiflexed to fit into a ski boot. On the left, she would ski without a prosthesis, but she might want to wear a stump socket to protect the stump and help keep it warm. For ski poles, she would use modified forearm crutches with small ski tips attached (called "outriggers"). Of course, she would need instructions in learning to use these new pieces of apparatus.

If skiing with a prosthesis proved to be uncomfortable, she could even learn to ski seated in a special frame mounted over a single ski called a "Monoski." This is what paraplegics use.

There are many centers where amputees can learn to participate in sports of all kinds. Children should be encouraged to join in. Parents often need support because it is natural for them to be protective, if not overprotective.

Case #10
Kooquious N. Berg

(Kooquious was named for a famous military ancestor, but was known to his friends as Cook'n)

Cook'n is a 12-year-old boy who went with his friend Ezekial for a hike into the hills of Colorado near his town. They discovered the entrance to an abandoned mine, and started to explore. Cook'n found an old blasting cap. Trying to take it apart he hit it with a rock. The resulting blast blew off both of his hands and blinded him at the same time.

By the way

Did you know that there are over one hundred million unexploded land mines in fields around the world left over from all of the wars? They have been the cause of tens of thousands of amputations, especially among farmers working their fields, as well as a huge number of accidents among children tending animals or playing with mines that they find.

Issues to ponder

1. What prostheses would you recommend?

2. What if Cook'n was not blind? Would you fit him with bilateral below-elbow prostheses?

3. What if he was not blind, lived on a farm in a remote part of Montana, and was needed by his family to do manual labor. He has a very difficult time getting to Billings to get prosthetic repairs, especially in the winter. What if he lived in Bangladesh?

Comments

1. Is a blind child likely to be able to use prosthetic hands? Remember that he will get no sensory feedback when he picks up an object in his prosthetic hand.

   Consider Krukenberg's operation. What is it? Here the skin and muscles between the radius and ulna are separated (rather like doing a syndactyly separation) so that the child can pinch between the two bones. He would be able to feel what he picks up even if he cannot see. The disadvantage of the operation is what some observers consider to be the unattractive cosmetic appearance of the result.

2. Yes, most people would fit him with bilateral below-elbow prostheses. He would be more likely to use them than if he was born without hands.

3. There is a growing realization that the potential functional benefits of a Krukenberg amputation may well outweigh the cosmetic disadvantages, especially if prosthetic services are not readily available, either because of geography or the limited resources in developing countries.

Case #11
Buckminster Q. Rogers

Buck is 10 years old. He was born with no arms, a little nub of a right lower extremity, and multiple congenital anomalies of his very short left lower extremity. He can move his left foot well under good control, but he can't reach his mouth with his foot, and he really doesn't have enough strength to hold onto a long handled spoon to feed himself. His father is a well-known and successful orthopaedic surgeon who has both financial resources and an understanding of the rehabilitation and bioengineering research going on around the world.

Issues to ponder

1. His father takes Buck to one center at which the staff suggest fitting Buck with bilateral upper extremity prostheses that are "switch controlled" by Buck's very effective left foot.

   If he were your son, would you agree to the effort?

2. The staff at another center suggest, as an alternative, fitting Buck to bilateral lower extremity prostheses: on the right, a modified hip disarticulation prosthesis, and on the left, a modified above-knee prosthesis. The left above-knee prosthesis would be modified to have a manual lock activated by Buck's left foot so that he would be stable when up walking, yet could bend his knee to sit down. Initially, both legs would be made quite short, so that Buck wouldn't feel afraid of falling over while he was learning to use the prostheses.

   If he were your son, would you agree to the effort?

3. You visit yet another center at which the staff try to convince you that an electric powered wheelchair is Buck's best device for "ambulation," meaning for traveling from one place to another. They also advise the father that the powered wheelchair could become the platform on which they could mount extra heavy-duty batteries that could power a "robotic" arm, which Buck could manipulate with his left foot, and also that they could fit the chair with a computer deck, which Buck could control with a small penlight laser attached to a head band. This way, Buck could use his computer to answer his phone, control household light switches, and even do his homework by modem.

   If he were your son, would you agree to the effort?

Comments

1. Just as with Amelia (see Case #6, page 29), the chance that Buck will use his prostheses is slim (the square root of zero, maybe?). Buck has very little surface area from which he can lose heat. Cover what little he has left with plastic, and he will find the prostheses not only cumbersome, but unbearably hot.

2. The energy expenditure for Buck to get up and walk would be enormous. Even if he could be fitted and taught how to walk, the prostheses would not be used to realistic functional advantage. Besides, with no arms, how is he going to get up on his feet from a chair?

3. All these things are currently possible, but the technology is in its infancy. If you head along this route, it would be most likely to succeed if each piece of equipment is added a step at time. A conventional prosthesis, attached to the body in the customary way, may not always be the best choice. The goal needs to be the replacement of lost function, and not necessarily the missing anatomic parts.

You are the R2 on

the Pediatric Orthopaedic service.

At 10:00 pm you are called by

the neonatal nursery to see

a new baby with a "deformed hand."

What are you going to say to the family?

Does that worry you?

Chapter 4

What Do You Say to the Family?

You are the first-year resident (R2) and have been on the Pediatric Orthopaedic service for 2 weeks. At 10:00 pm you are called by the neonatal nursery and asked to consult on a new baby with a "deformed hand."

Will you say:

a. "I'll bring Dr. Attends by tomorrow after the operating room."

b. "I'm not on hand call; better call the plastics guys."

c. "I'll be right over; how do I get there?"

The answer is "c." Yes, it ***is*** that urgent! Put yourself in the place of the parents who have just experienced a sudden silence in the delivery room, followed by something, such as the baby's being wrapped quickly and whisked away or the nurse saying sotto voce, "Were you expecting a congenital deformity?" Some of these parents literally believe their baby is dead. All of this is the result of the rarity of these occurrences in any single delivery room and the fact that no one present knows what to say.

Although you may not think you know what to say either, you can still do something extraordinarily important: you can influence the way in which the parents perceive their new baby, and you can alleviate significant human suffering by following these simple principles:

1. Go see the baby and the parents as soon as possible.
2. Examine the entire baby (think syndrome, see Chapter 3).
3. Take the baby with you if it's not already with the parents, and go see them. Let one of them hold the baby.

4. Sit down—to relax them, and so that you do not to talk down to them in any way.

5. Admire the beautiful baby. Play with it a little, get it to respond to you. It is a normal baby who happens to have some differences (almost always; if you are concerned that it is not really a "normal" baby, admire it generally, and later discuss your concerns with the pediatric orthopaedist or pediatrician. Of the many syndromes involving limb deficiencies, only a few include mental retardation).

6. Describe in simple terms what the situation is. "The thigh bone did not fully develop," or "one of the bones in her arm is missing." (Try to avoid using words that sound bad: "deformity," "malformation," "abnormality," and so forth.) Emphasize that there was nothing they did (or did not do) that caused this situation.

7. Say that you will call the pediatric orthopaedist, who can give them more details.

Chapter 5

What Do You Say to the Chart?

Terminology Issues

In the clinic and at meetings we all talk with each other easily and understandably about "a patient with an absent tibia" or a "congenital BE" (a below-elbow limb deletion). But the details of the exact anatomy of congenital deficiencies are important for treatment decisions, and for later chart review for comparison of apples with apples, etc., for research purposes.

Several systems of terminology have been and are still in use, in the United States and in other countries (Outline 1). However, hemimelia, ectromelia, peromelia, dysmelia, and other terms mean different things to different people.

In 1973, an international committee established by the International Society for Prosthetics and Orthotics (ISPO) first met, and eventually produced an International Terminology accepted by the World Health Organization and the International Standards Organization in 1988. It even has an official number. Now all countries and all languages can use the same scheme for describing congenital limb differences.

The basics of the International Terminology are simple:

- **Name the side** (L, R, or B).

- **Decide if the deficiency is longitudinal or transverse.** Transverse resembles a surgical amputation, with no remaining distal part; longitudinal is anything else. (Small remnants of rudimentary fingers or toes ("nubbins") do not count as remaining distal parts.)

- **If transverse, say so and name the level of loss:** "left transverse forearm deficiency, proximal third."

- **If longitudinal, say so and name the missing bones as nouns,** modified by partial or total (absence), from proximal to distal: "right longitudinal deficiency, radius, total; rays 1&2, partial." ("Ray" refers, more briefly, to a metacarpal or metatarsal and all of its associated phalanges.)

Additional embellishments that you may use include hypoplastic, fused, and so forth.

Obviously we are not going to speak in the clinic about the "new kid with right longitudinal deficiency, femur partial, proximal one third, fibula total, tarsus partial, rays four and five total." We will speak about the new kid with the PFFD with absent fibula and a three-toed foot. But, encountering the former in the chart, when you are the person comparing all the children with PFFD who had knee fusions done at a particular hospital to those who had van Nes rotationplasties, will make you very happy.

Outline 1
Some Synonyms Used in Past Literature

Shared terms

melia: Greek root for "limb"

amelia: "a" = absence, "melia" = the limb; therefore, absence of limb

phocomelia: literally, a limb like a seal (ie, the marine animal) used for a hand or foot attached directly to the trunk

Frantz and O'Rahilly (United States)

hemimelia: literally half a limb; in practice a longitudinal deficiency

meromelia: partial limb; synonym for hemimelia, used by etymologic sticklers

intercalary: a part missing out of the middle, eg, absent radius with five-rayed hand

terminal: a longitudinal deficiency with a long bone and its related distal part missing totally, eg, absent fibula and missing fourth and fifth rays

European

peromelia: peros = maimed (Greek)

ectromelia: ectro = miscarriage (Greek). A combining form signifying the congenital absence of a part

dysmelia: Greek root. A combining form signifying difficult, painful, bad, disordered, abnormal

Appendix

What Should I See When I Look at a Prosthesis?

This is not intended to provide a complete course in prosthetics; hence, it is added as an appendix. However, it is provided as an overview so that you will have some basis to work with when you start to see patients with prostheses.

A prosthesis is an extension of the body replacing some function that is missing. Keep in mind that cosmetic appearance can be an important function in many people's minds.

The specifics that need to be considered are particular to a given level of amputation. Because the prostheses of the lower and upper extremities are so fundamentally different, they will be discussed in separate sections. Each section is further subdivided by the level at which the amputation or limb deletion has occurred. Each level of prosthetic need will be reviewed in a standard format:

A. The working end

- Power
- Power control

B. Positioning

- Extensions
- Joints and joint control

C. Load transfer

D. Security

- Suspension
- Torque control

When looking at a prosthesis, you need to consider:

A. The working end

This, after all, is what the prosthesis is trying to replace. In the lower extremity, this is usually a foot (unless you are dealing, for example, with a special swimming model in which a flipper might be used). In the upper extremity, the working end is usually something that allows for grasp, ie, a hook or a hand, and commonly is called a terminal device.

Power In the upper extremity, the working end usually has moving parts. These parts require some form of power to activate them. This power may be provided by the patient's own body muscles (using a cable if the body muscle used is at some distance from the working end). Alternatively, power can be provided by electric motors.

In the past, compressed carbon dioxide has been used, but it currently is not favored because the canisters were bulky, heavy, and not readily recharged.

Power Control Any time external power is used, there is need for controlling the power. In the case of an electric motor, the power can be switched on and off manually. This might be used for a child born with a short arm that has one digit at the end that could be used to turn a switch on and off.

Alternatively, and more commonly, the power can be controlled by myoelectric impulses (created by the voluntary activity of muscles underneath the skin), which are picked up through the skin by smooth electrodes that protrude slightly from the inside surface of the socket.

B. Positioning

In order to put the working end in a place where the desired work can be done most advantageously, there is usually a need for extension(s) to replace the length lost from the amputation or congenital deletion. Furthermore, there may be a need for one or more joints to position the working end to the best advantage.

Extensions Extensions may be composed of a skeleton of simple pipes underneath a shaped foam cover, ie, "Endoskeletal." This construction provides a modular and thus easily modified system and can result in a cosmetically appealing soft outer shape. Older children appreciate this construction, and appreciation is not restricted to the girls.

Younger children, who are less likely to be fiscally responsible, can tear up foam cosmetic covers at an astonishing rate. For them, extensions are usually more wisely constructed of the same hard material that the sockets are made of and are sometimes referred to as "Exoskeletal."

Joints Whenever there are joints, they may or may not need power to activate or control their motion. Controls may be simple locks to prevent unwanted motion (eg, a knee lock in a young child who is a new above-knee prosthesis wearer), or they may rely on careful alignment of the joints to use the force of body weight to keep a joint from collapsing during stance phase of gait. To explain this why don't you stand up. Now lean forward at your waist and reach down to grasp one of your patellas between your thumb and your index. When you are leaning forward, you can wobble your patella from side to side. What does this tell you? It tells you that your quadriceps isn't doing any work. You are actually standing up without using your quadriceps. That is because your center of gravity falls in front of your knee joint and so gravity is working to extend your knee. The ligaments at the back of the knee are preventing your knee from hyperextending, thereby supporting your weight. Now with your thumb and index wobbling your patella, gradually flex your knees. You will see that you come to a point when your knee is flexed about 10 degrees to 25 degrees when you can't move your patella. That's the point at which the quadriceps start doing their work. In exactly the same way, if a child's prosthesis is aligned so that the center of gravity falls anterior to the axis of the knee joint, and the knee joint is contructed so that hyperextension can't take place, then the knee joint will not buckle. Look for what provides the joint control.

C. Load transfer

The forces from the working end need to be transferred to the rest of the body. The mechanism of load transfer is generally a somewhat tubular socket that fits over the residual limb. The transfer of the loads may be as simple as the friction between the socket and the patient's skin or it may be more complex, involving selected areas of high-pressure loading in locations, such as the ischial tuberosity, where the skin can tolerate this high load.

D. Security

Imagine getting up from a bar stool and having your leg fall off. It could prove to be very embarrassing. Or suppose you were standing around and turned quickly to your right and your prosthesis stayed facing the wrong direction. Not only might you be embarrassed; you might fall.

Suspension To prevent the prosthesis from slipping off, some mechanism must be provided to secure it to the patient's body.

Torque control Some mechanism also may be required to prevent the prosthesis from spinning around on the stump. Not uncommonly, the mechanism that prevents a prosthesis from slipping off also prevents the prosthesis from twisting on the stump.

Lower Extremity

Partial Foot

These amputations or deletions certainly are seen in children, and they may be at any of the standard levels: ray deletions, transmetatarsal, Chopart or Lisfranc levels, or even mixed medial to lateral, especially if congenital. However, they are less common and can usually be taken care of with a shoe filler, a partial foot prosthesis, or sometimes an ankle-foot orthosis. Longer feet do well in sneakers or other high-top shoes. We will say no more than that.

Syme's Amputation

Syme originally described an ankle disarticulation. In adults, current usage is for removal of the malleoli. In children, however, joint disarticulation with the cartilage left in place is the preferred technique to eliminate the possibility of bony overgrowth.

A. The working end

This is usually the standard SACH (solid ankle cushion heel) foot. The presence of the cushion at the heel simulates ankle plantarflexion on heel strike and allows for some simulated inversion and eversion. The cushion needs to be softer (less dense) for small children. The absence of an ankle joint means one less thing to be repaired. Fancier energy-storing feet can be used in athletic achievers who have money to burn, however, the options are increasing and the costs decreasing.

Power to swing the prosthesis is provided by the patient's own lower extremity muscles.

Power control is not needed because no external power is needed.

B. Positioning

Extensions All that is needed is a simple prolongation of the socket to the level of the junction with the foot.

Joints None are needed; therefore, Joint control is not needed.

C. Load transfer

This is end bearing through the soft tissue of the heel pad, which has been brought around at the end of the stump. Posterior migration of the heel pad because of retained attachments to the heel cord seldom proves to be a problem in children because the skin over the end of the stump will thicken to accommodate load bearing.

D. Security

Suspension This is provided by a tight fit at the narrower diameter of the tibia, just proximal to the malleoli. In adults, some surgeons remove the malleoli so that an unsightly bulge does not occur in the prosthesis at the ankle level. In children, the tibia on the deformed side usually grows more slowly than the tibia on the normal side. Therefore, the bulge at the malleolar level gradually migrates proximally, which really means that the opposite leg is growing more. This migration results in the bulge on the amputated side being accommodated at the level of the calf on the normal side so that it passes unnoticed. Leaving the malleoli on provides a more secure suspension.

The wider end of the distal tibia can be inserted into a prosthesis either through a window with a cover in the prosthesis or by the use of a soft liner that is constricted at the level of the tibia, just proximal to the malleoli.

Torque control This is obtained by the shape of the distal tibia, which is wider from medial-to-lateral than from front-to-back.

Below the Knee (BK)

A. The working end

This is commonly a SACH foot.

Power from another source is not needed.

Power control is not needed because external power is not needed.

B. Positioning

Extensions The distance between the bottom of the socket for a below-knee amputation and the foot can be filled by either a solid block continuation of the socket to meet the ankle connection or an endoskeletal pipe. The segment is very short; therefore, a soft cosmetic cover is not an advantage to the patient.

Joints None are needed; therefore, Joint control is not needed.

C. Load transfer

The forces from the floor go up to the socket, and the transfer to the stump is through the oblique surfaces of the medial and lateral flares of the proximal tibia and to some extent through the infrapatellar ligament area. Because of the sloping surfaces of the proximal tibia, the natural tendency is for the stump to sink down into the socket. As it sinks, the stump shifts posteriorly. The stump is prevented from sinking by having a posterior pressure area between the heads of the gastrocnemius muscle and by holding the knee slightly flexed. Because of the common sensitivity of the end of the stump in a transtibial amputation, a soft pad usually is added to the inside of the socket at its distal end.

D. Security

Suspension This is frequently achieved by the use of a circumferential strap proximal to the femoral condyles, or often now, a neoprene (or other similar material) 'suspension sleeve,' rolled up from the prosthesis onto the limb. Alternatively, the socket can be made to extend proximal to the femoral condyles and can then be held in place by a wedge-shaped pad inserted between the upper medial part of the socket and the superior surface of the medial femoral condyle.

Torque control This is managed by the shape of the tibia in that the proximal tibia is broader from medial to lateral than from anterior to posterior.

Knee Disarticulation

A. The working end

This is commonly a SACH foot.

Power from another source is not needed.

Power control is not needed because external power is not needed.

B. Positioning

Extensions An extension is needed from below the knee joint down to the foot. A piece of pipe can be used as an endoskeletal unit from the bottom line of the knee joint down to the foot, or a separate solid shin segment can be fabricated as with a below-knee prosthesis (see above).

Joint A knee joint, which requires approximately 7 cm of space, is now needed. Therefore, the knee heights will be at different levels. The asymmetry of knee levels is not an issue if the child has a congenital anomaly whereby the femur on the knee-disarticulation side is particularly short. An alternative is the use of outside knee joints; however, these are not as cosmetically appealing and can readily tear the trouser leg. Proper planning can allow for a distal femoral epiphysiodesis to provide symmetric knee heights at skeletal maturity.

Joint control The control of the knee joint is obtained by aligning the knee joint with the center of gravity anterior to the axis of the prosthetic knee joint. Therefore, in stance, the knee is safely locked into full extension by the force of gravity.

C. Load transfer

This is "end bearing" from the bottom of the socket to the broad area of skin overlying the distal femoral condyles.

D. Security

Suspension Because the distal femoral condyles are wider than the adjacent diaphysis of the femur, the socket can be made self-suspending. This is done most easily by having an inner liner. This inner liner has a split (both medially and laterally) such that the broad end of the femur can pass by the narrow isthmus in the soft liner. Once the femur is in its proper place in the liner, the liner is pushed into the socket. The liner is now unable to expand and, therefore, the femoral condyles are held in place.

Torque control Torque is controlled by the shape of the femoral condyles, which are broader from medial to lateral than they are from anterior to posterior.

Above the Knee (AK)

A. The working end

This is commonly a SACH foot.

Power from another source is not needed.

Power control is not needed because external power is not needed.

B. Positioning

Extensions Extensions are needed as in a knee-disarticulation prosthesis (see above) except that shorter lengths of femoral stump may require an extension between the socket and the knee joint as well as between the knee joint and the foot.

Joint and **joint control** *See above under* Knee Disarticulation.

C. Load transfer

Currently there are two systems used to transfer loaded forces. The more classic approach has been that of ischial bearing, in which the upper end of the socket is flared posteriorly, and the patient essentially sits on the flare with the ischial tuberosity resting on this flare. To keep the ischial tuberosity from sliding over the anterior edge of the flare and allowing the stump to sink into the socket, counter pressure from an anterior direction is needed to keep the ischial tuberosity posteriorly on the flare. This anterior pressure area is formed over Scarpa's triangle.

A more recent approach is that of "Ischial Containment," in which the ischium is fitted inside the socket and the medial-lateral dimension is narrowed; load transfer takes place primarily by the friction between the socket and the patient's skin.

D. Security

Suspension This is characteristically attained by the use of a belt that goes from the anterior part of the prosthesis across the front of the torso, around the opposite ilium (just below the iliac crest and above the greater trocanter), and then around posteriorly to the posterior lateral margin of the socket. The belt characteristically is called a Silesian belt. If the waist contours are not well-defined, a modified Silesian belt may be used instead. This one is a circumferential belt with two oblique straps, one going anteriorly from about the midline and directed inferiorly and laterally to the anterior lip of the prosthesis, and then a similar posterior strap going obliquely from the strap down and laterally to the posterolateral part of the socket. If such suspension is not practical, a belt is provided that has shoulder straps (like a parachute harness). From this belt, oblique suspension straps are provided. Another option is an elastic, neoprene, or gel-like suspension sleeve which can encompass the socket and extend up around the waist.

Suction suspension may be used. Remember when you were young and foolish enough to be talked into sticking your finger into a coke bottle only to find it very hard to remove? The principle is the same. The inferior end of the above-knee socket is fitted with a one-way valve, so that when the stump is pushed into the socket (in point of fact, the stump is drawn down into the socket using a stump wrap) and the valve cap put into place, the stump is held. This suspension has the virtue of eliminating straps, but is not frequently used in children. Suction suspension requires a very snug fit. Because children are growing, a persisting snug fit over many months is not easily maintained, although the use of a flexible socket may help with this. Hot weather with excessive sweating makes suction suspension more difficult to accomplish.

Torque control Torque is controlled by the use of the suspension techniques described above.

Hip Disarticulation

A. The working end

This is commonly a SACH foot.

Power from another source is not needed.

Power control is not needed because external power is not needed.

B. Positioning

Extensions Now two extensions are required: one from the hip joint down to the knee and another from the knee joint down to the foot. These extensions are most commonly endoskeletal.

Joints Two joints are needed: one to replace the hip and one to replace the knee. At the hip, the joint is hinged anteriorly (opens posteriorly) to allow for hip flexion in swing phase and for sitting. The knee joint is the same as described for an above-knee amputee.

Joint control Control for the hip joint is attained by having the line of weightbearing posterior to the joint axis so that, in stance, the weight of the body closes the hip hinge. Control for the knee joint is the same as described for the above-knee amputee.

C. Load transfer

This requires a socket that fits around the lower torso. The loads are transferred to the ischium and the surrounding soft tissues as the patient sits within the socket.

D. Security

Suspension The socket is molded over the iliac crests to hold the prosthesis in place.

Torque control Torque is controlled by the pelvis enclosed within the socket, which is broader from medial-to-lateral than from anterior-to-posterior.

Hemipelvectomy

A. The working end

This is commonly a SACH foot.

Power from another source is not needed.

Power control is not needed because external power is not needed.

B. Positioning

This is the same as with the hip disarticulation.

C. Load transfer

Here the problem is different from the hip disarticulation in that there is no ischial tuberosity. Load bearing is by hydrostatic containment of soft tissues and by friction between the socket and the patient's skin over the lower abdominal wall and under the ribs.

D. Security

Suspension This is achieved by molding the socket around the opposite iliac crest.

Torque control This is achieved by getting a mold around the opposite iliac wing.

The Wheelchair

Do not forget that the wheelchair is also a prosthesis, an extension of the body that replaces a missing function.

Fitting the wheelchair into the same schema as the above prostheses may be a bit absurd, but we will try it in order for you to keep in mind that a wheelchair may be the best option for ambulation (ie, getting from point A to point B) for some children with multiple limb deficiencies.

A. The working end

This is the wheels.

Power If a child has no upper extremities, power may be needed, usually from electric motors that use large car batteries mounted to the wheelchair chassis.

Controls The power, if needed, is usually controlled by a joystick mounted at a site convenient to what the child has left that the child can voluntarily control. This may be a hand or finger, a lower extremity residual, or the neck.

B. Positioning

Extensions These may include a balanced arm feeder, a table, and communications equipment.

Joints These may include a folding bottom for transport, a reclining back, and removable arms for transfer.

C. Load transfer

Occasionally, special cushioning may be required to decrease the likelihood of the child's developing pressure sores under the ischial tuberositites. This is most likely needed for a child who lacks sensation below the waist.

D. Security

Suspension Use a safety belt! Children like to race their wheelchairs every bit as much as adults like to race their cars from stop lights.

Torque control This is not needed.

Upper Extremity

Hands and Fingers

Although prostheses are sometimes provided for loss at this level, they usually are more a hindrance to sensation and activity and generally are not used except for special events at which cosmetic appearance is primary.

Transcarpal/Transmetacarpal

Frequently, nothing is used. Sometimes, if there are carpal bones that can be actively moved by the patient, a post is provided against which the carpal bones can be pressed for prehension. This post is an extension of a cuff that fits around the distal forearm.

A. The working end

Power is provided by the patient's own wrist volar flexors, which are used to force the residual wrist against the opposition post of the prosthesis.

Power control is the patient's own proprioception.

B. Positioning

Extensions None are needed.

Joints Because the width of grasp needed with an opposition post varies (eg, for objects ranging from a slender pen to larger objects, such as a drinking glass), the post may be hinged at preset intervals.

Joint control The selection of the preset interval is made with the other hand.

C. Load transfer

This is by friction between the forearm mold and the skin of the forearm.

D. Security

Suspension This is by straps around the forearm.

Torque control This is from the same straps and is provided because the forearm is broader from medial-to-lateral than anterior-to-posterior.

Below Elbow (BE) Including Wrist Disarticulation

A. The working end

This is usually either a hook or hand. A hook has the advantage of simplicity and durability. In addition, it occupies a small visual area and does not obstruct the wearer from being able to see what is being picked up.

In spite of what you may imagine after watching "That's Incredible" on television, a mechanical hand does not have the freedom of motion that a normal hand does. A mechanical hand usually is constructed with an index and long finger that are fused together and move as a single unit against a thumb that can move only in the same plane as the opposing fingers. Grasp is achieved by pinch (commonly called a "three jawed chuck"). The hand is covered by a plastic cosmetic glove. The advantages of a hand over a hook are primarily cosmetic, but that is a most powerful appeal. The disadvantages are that the glove is readily torn; the hand itself is less durable and is more expensive.

There are other terminal devices, (TD's) principally the CAPP TD, which has a moving "thumb" that moves against a solid block palm.

Terminal devices can be broadly grouped into those that are voluntary opening and those that are voluntary closing. Voluntary opening devices are kept closed by springs or elastics and require some power to open them up. Voluntary closing devices are kept in an open position and require force to close them. With voluntary opening devices, the wearer does not need constant force to hold an object; the spring or elastic does that. Therefore, they are less tiring. Voluntary closing devices have the advantage that a wearer can vary the amount of force applied to an object that is being pinched. Those who prefer voluntary closing devices feel that an element of proprioceptive feedback is gained.

In the past, voluntary opening devices have been the overwhelming standard. More recently, there has been renewed interest in voluntary closing devices, that can be fitted with a lock, that can hold a terminal device closed.

Power The power needed to activate a terminal device can be either body muscles or electric motors. The body power is transmitted from the power source (the opposite shoulder's ability to be moved anteriorly) by a cable to the terminal device. This cable runs from a loop worn around the opposite shoulder, across the back, behind the triceps (where it is anchored so the cable does not pop in front of the elbow), along the posterolateral aspect of the forearm, and then to the terminal device. Moving the scapula forward increases the distance from the proximal end of the cable to the terminal device. Because the cable cannot stretch, the terminal device is opened (on a voluntary opening device). Body power has the advantages of rapid motion and the absence of battery failure.

Conversely, an electric motor can be placed within the forearm segment of the below-elbow prosthesis. Batteries may be placed in the forearm segment. If the forearm stump is long, this leaves little room for both motor and batteries, so the battery pack would need to be worn elsewhere on the body. Electric power does mean the potential for battery run down, which is less of a problem than in the past but can still be a problem. However, the use of electric power obviates the need for harness straps.

Power control In an electrically driven terminal device, power control is commonly by myoelectric impulses. Characteristically, the electrodes are placed over the proximal extensor and flexor muscles of the forearm. A surface electromyographic signal from a voluntary twitch of the appropriate muscle turns on the battery that energizes the electric motor, which in turn drives gears that activate the fingers. Sometimes, control is achieved by using switches that are manually activated (eg, by a shrug of the shoulder, the chin, or a minimal pull on a harness system). Such switch systems are more likely to be used in children with multiple limb deficiencies.

B. Positioning

Extensions From the socket to the hand, an extension is required. This extension is usually hollow and may be the housing for the motor and batteries as described above.

Joints A wrist positioning joint for volar and dorsal flexion as well as pronation and supination may be included. However, the length of the stump and the added complexity may obviate the advantage of having the added flexibility.

Joint control The control of the joint is by the opposite hand to preposition the prosthetic terminal device to the appropriate attitude.

C. Load transfer

This is skin friction between the socket and the skin enhanced by the conical shape of the proximal forearm.

D. Security

Suspension This may be provided by molding the upper end of the socket above the olecranon and around the humeral condyles. This method is used more characteristically with very short below-elbow stumps. More commonly, suspension is by either the strap that goes up the back of the arm to the opposite shoulder ring or, in myoelectric prostheses (for which no shoulder strap is used), a rubberized sleeve may hold the prosthesis in place.

Torque control This is provided by friction between the socket and the prosthesis and is always a bit of a problem. This problem is made worse in patients with shorter stumps. The medial-to-lateral socket molding of the socket helps.

Elbow Disarticulation

This is managed basically in the same way as an above-elbow amputation, except that the arm can be suspended over the humeral condyles, and the shape of the distal humerus can be used to provide more rotational control.

Above Elbow (AE)

A. The working end

The choice of terminal devices and use of **Power** and **Power control** are as stated above for below-elbow prostheses.

B. Positioning

Extensions This may require an extension between the socket and the elbow joint as well as one between the elbow joint and the terminal device.

Joints An elbow joint is now required. This can be controlled by either body power or by electric power. In the body powered construction, the elbow joint has a multiposition lock.

Joint control The control end of the elbow lock is attached to a strap that goes across the front of the shoulder joint. The upper end of this strap is attached to the main figure of 8 harness that loops over both shoulders posteriorly. Abduction of the ipsilateral shoulder increases the distance between the elbow joint and the front of the shoulder, essentially pulling on the lock strap. At that point, the elbow is free to go through its full range of motion. By moving the opposite shoulder anteriorly (pulling on the cable that opens the terminal device), the elbow flexes. Flexion occurs because the cable passes in front of the axis of the elbow joint, and the terminal device does not open because it is stiffer than the force required to flex the elbow. When the elbow is in the desired position, the ipsilateral shoulder is again abducted to activate the elbow lock and hold the elbow at the degree of flexion that the wearer has selected. At that point, forward motion of the opposite shoulder (ie, again pulling on the terminal device control cable) will activate the terminal device because the elbow is now locked.

C. Load transfer

This is by friction between the skin and the socket.

D. Security

Suspension This is achieved through the straps that circle the two shoulders.

Torque Control There is no adequate prosthetic means of controlling torque in an above-elbow prosthesis. If the prosthesis is held in full extension and the shoulder flexed to 90° in front of the body, there is no problem with torque. If, however, the elbow is flexed at all, the weight of the terminal device will spin the prosthesis on the axis of the stump. It is therefore very hard for an above-elbow prosthesis wearer to raise the prosthetic hand much above the shoulder. This problem may be decreased with careful molding of the socket in the anterior deltopectoral groove and posteriorly. A short right-angle osteotomy of the distal humerus can provide a prominence around which the socket is fitted. This procedure does allow torque control. It also can be used for suspension. In children, however, the right-angle osteotomy has been less successful because it tends to remodel into a straight bone.

Shoulder Disarticulation

These prostheses are used mostly for cosmetic purposes.
(See page 10—***poor gadget tolerance.***)

Forequarter Amputation

As with shoulder disarticulation, prostheses at this level usually are discarded as being hot and bothersome. They are generally reserved for cosmetic benefits. A simple molded shoulder pad held in place by a strap across the chest can help clothes fit better.

Some Handy Resources

These are for you

Fisk JR, Introduction to the child amputee, in Bowker JH, Michael JW (eds): *AAOS Atlas of Limb Prosthetics: Surgical, Prosthetic, and Rehabilitation Principles.* St. Louis, MO, Mosby Year Book, 1992, pp 731–734.

Goldberg MJ: *The Dysmorphic Child: An Orthopaedic Perspective.* New York, NY, Raven Press, 1987.

Herring JA, Birch JC (eds): *The Child With a Limb Deficiency.* Rosemont, IL, American Academy of Orthopaedic Surgeons, 1998.

Herring JA, Cummings DR: The limb-deficient child, in Morrissy RT, Weinstein SL (eds): *Lovell and Winter's Pediatric Orthopaedics,* ed 4. Philadelphia, PA, Lippincott-Raven, 1996, pp 1137–1180.

Jones KL (ed): *Smith's Recognizable Patterns of Human Malformation,* ed 5. Philadelphia, PA, WB Saunders, 1997.

Krahn GL, Hallum A, Kime C: Are there good ways to give "bad news"? *Pediatrics* 1993;91:578–582.

O'Leary H: *Bold Tracks: Teaching Adaptive Skiing,* ed 3. Winter Park, CO, National Sports Center for the Disabled, Johnson Books, 1994.

These are for the children's families

SuperKids, newsletter, 60 Clyde Street, Newton MA 02160

This free (donations appreciated) newsletter is put out two to three times per year. It is a well-done, informative publication with featured picture stories of children with limb differences, letters from kids and families, and pertinent news items.

The same people also publish a *Directory of Families,* including information about the limb difference, with addresses and phone numbers, to facilitate connections among those with similar situations. $5 for families; $10 for clinics; revised every 1 to 2 years.

Children with Limb Loss: A Handbook for Families (Birth to 5 years)

Children with Limb Loss: A Handbook for Families (6 to 12 years)

Adolescents with Limb Loss: A Handbook for Adolescents and Their Families

Children with Hand Differences: A Guide for Families (also available in Spanish)

Children with Limb Loss: A Handbook for Teachers

All of the above titles are available from
Area Child Amputee Center
235 Wealthy Street SE
Grand Rapids, MI 49503
616-454-7988

On the Internet

www.amputee-coalition.org	National Limb Loss Information Center
www.nscd.org	National Sports Center for the Disabled
users.southeast.net/~bbaughn/childamp.htm	I-CAN! Information-Child Amputee Network

Good Luck!